THE HIGH-ENERGY FACTOR

THE HIGH-ENERGY FACTOR

*The No-Diet Way to
Slimness and Health Through
Natural Exercise*

Dr. Bernard Gutin
with Gail Kessler

*Random House
New York*

Grateful acknowledgment is made to Cambridge University Press and to the William C. Brown Company Publishers for permission to reprint a figure from Fitness for Life: An Individualized Approach, *2nd ed., by Philip E. Allsen et al. © 1975, 1976, 1980 by William C. Brown Company Publishers, Dubuque, Iowa. Adapted from a figure by J.V.G.A. Durnin and J. Womersley published in* British Journal of Nutrition, *vol. 32, 1974, p. 95, Cambridge University Press. Reprinted by permission of the publishers.*

Library of Congress Cataloging in Publication Data
Gutin, Bernard, 1934–
   The High-energy factor.
   Bibliography: p.
   Includes index.
   1. Reducing diets. 2. Health. I. Kessler, Gail, 1937–   '
II. Title.
RM222.2.G85   1983   613.2'5   82-13353
ISBN 0-394-52548-5

Manufactured in the United States of America

98765432

First Edition

To Chelley, Glenn and Linda

Better to hunt in fields, for health unbought,
Than fee the doctor for a nauseous draught.
The wise, for cure, on exercise depend;
God never made his work for man to mend.

—John Dryden, 1631–1700

Introduction

When people find out what I do for a living (teach and do research on exercise physiology and nutrition), they generally react in one of three ways: they start apologizing for their own lack of fitness, they ask for advice on their own exercise and eating habits, or they ask what I do to stay in shape. People who are aware of the benefits of physical activity often express envy of the fact that I get paid to keep myself and others healthy! Over the years, many friends and acquaintances have come to think of me as their personal exercise guru. I've enjoyed advising them, and hope to go one doing so; but a couple of years ago it occurred to me that it might be helpful, not only to them but to many other people trying to lose weight, keep it off, and stay healthy, if I were to collect what I know about exercise and its interactions with nutrition into a book.

At the same time, several other factors helped me make the decision to write this book. For one thing, many patients at the weight control center where I am director of physiology had been finding that while dieting could help them lose weight temporarily, the only thing that made long-term success possible for them was a permanent change to a more active lifestyle, and they urged me to help them share this discovery with as many people as possible. In addition, graduate students in my seminars at Teachers College, Columbia University, who along with me had been analyzing all the literature on the role of diet and exercise in weight control, were becoming convinced that recent research findings were so important that they should be summarized and interpreted for the public. Finally, one of my friends, freelance writer Gail Kessler, was excited enough by the new research to want to help bring it to the attention of a public that is constantly bombarded by weight-loss plans having two factors in common: they're based on dieting, and they don't work.

In recent years, many physicians, nutritionists and psychologists have become so discouraged by the dismal long-term success rate of dieting that they have begun to call obesity an incurable disease. At the same time, research by a diverse group of professionals, including exercise physiologists, has pointed to increased energy expenditure as a crucial element in long-term maintenance of weight loss: the "high-energy factor." My own clinical experience at a hospital-based weight control center has supported this idea. The clinical reports and research (some from my own laboratory) continue to accumulate even as this book is being completed. It's rare that a week goes by without some item about the effects of exercise on both weight control and health appearing in the newspapers.

Though information continues to pile up, the basic conclusions are quite clear, and it's unlikely that future research will alter them in any fundamental way:

- The cause of obesity is much more likely to be a sedentary (low-energy) lifestyle than excessive calorie intake.
- The body resists unnatural dieting, which it perceives as starvation, and tries to restore the lost weight at the first opportunity.
- Increasing your energy expenditure through natural exercise— that is, living a high-energy lifestyle—allows you to lose weight gradually and *permanently* while eating enough to satisfy hunger and meet the body's nutritional needs.

High-energy living, in the final analysis, is simply a recapturing of some of the healthy habits of our distant ancestors: adequate intake of nutritious foods and active *use* of our bodies.

Here's what the book includes:

- An analysis of the most recent scientific information on the interactions of exercise, nutrition, weight control, and health, including the reasons why dieting is unnatural and resisted by the body, while increased activity is natural and beneficial.
- Specific guidance on how to take charge of your weight and well-being through increased energy expenditure, including

strategies for both the very sedentary and those moving on to high levels of fitness. There are special pointers for women, and guidelines for the very obese, the young, the old, diabetics, and people with cardiac or pulmonary disease.

· An explanation of how high-energy living provides protection from most of our society's major health problems, both physiological (e.g., heart disease) and psychological (e.g., depression).

· Optimal nutrition for health, physical performance, and weight control.

· Suggestions for societal changes to facilitate high-energy living on a large scale.

· Extensive tables giving calories used in various activities, calories in and composition of many foods, amounts of weight that can be lost by increased exercise, and the number of weeks it takes to lose ten, thirty, or fifty pounds by introducing the high-energy factor into your life.

The close link of physical activity to joy is easily seen in children at play. As we become adults, however, we often leave much of our youthful activity—and the joy that goes along with it—behind us. With the serious business of adulthood comes a thickening of our waistlines and a weakening of our muscles, making physical exertion difficult and reducing our activity even more. If we allow this process to continue, we don't look good, we don't feel good, and we are more susceptible to many of life's ills. But the millions of people who are discovering, or rediscovering, the joy of movement are living proof that adulthood doesn't have to be a time of increased girth and decreased vitality. By following the guidelines offered in this book, you can join the growing numbers of high-energy people who eat with gusto rather than guilt, who view their bodies with pride instead of shame, and who undertake physical challenges with confidence in place of doubt.

I believe that my particular combination of scholarly, clinical and personal experience, along with the literary talents of Gail Kessler, have resulted in a comprehensive guide to a high-energy lifestyle that will enable you to attain permanent slimness and dynamic health.

—Bernard Gutin
November 1982

Acknowledgments

When a book touches on so much of one's professional and personal life, as this one does, it is impossible to acknowledge all the people who contributed in some way. I hope that all my unmentioned friends and colleagues will not think me ungrateful for their help and support over the years. I must thank publicly my wife, Chelley, who has for twenty-five years been a major influence on everything I've done. As a university professor, I must mention the influence of my students and colleagues in shaping my thinking and collaborating on much of the research mentioned in these pages. More specific thanks are due to colleagues who read and commented on parts of the manuscript: Isobel Contento, Ph.D., David Pargman, Ph.D., Michael Sacks, M.D., and Karen Segal, Ed.D. Whatever literary qualities the manuscript has are due to the excellent work of Gail Kessler and Nancy Inglis. For the charts in chapter 5 I must thank Jim Gold. And Tom Rotell has given me many hours of valuable advice during our runs.

Contents

THE HIGH-ENERGY FACTOR

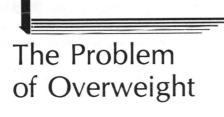

The Problem
of Overweight

I give many talks to adult groups, and often ask my audiences how many of them are watching their weight by restricting their eating. The first time I did this, I was amazed to see that nearly all the people present raised their hands. By this time I've come to expect it. Americans are definitely a nation of weightwatchers. Even those of us who, to judge by our appearance, don't have a weight problem still feel the need to be eternally vigilant about overeating lest we put on those two or three or five unwanted pounds.*

Why are so many Americans preoccupied with their weight?

For one thing, we place a very high value on personal attractiveness in our society, especially for women, and slenderness is thought to be attractive, while fat is considered ugly.

Second, the fat person is usually viewed as lacking in self-control, weak, at the mercy of his or her appetite—and in a nation that stresses individual enterprise and self-reliance, that's an unenviable way to be.

And finally, there are important health reasons for being slender.

---

*If you would like some guidelines as to how much you should weigh, see the Appendix.

Overweight (over*fat,* actually) has been linked to many of the major killer diseases of our time.

So what do we do to solve our weight problem? We think we are overweight because we eat too much, so we try to eat less. We take diet pills to reduce our appetites and we go on a variety of reducing diets. A huge industry has been created around Americans' weight consciousness. Yet a look at the caloric intake of Americans over the past eighty years or so shows that our average food intake has *dropped* more than 10 percent from what it was at the turn of the century. *Americans are currently eating fewer calories* than we were in 1900 —yet more of us are overweight than ever before.† Why?*

For the answer, we have to go back a good many thousands of years. For most of mankind's history, food was far from plentiful. In fact, survival depended on the ability to store food efficiently in the body when food was available, against the time when it would be scarce. It was important to utilize as little energy as possible during hard times, to avoid using up stored food. A lowered metabolic rate in times of scarcity contributed to the conservation of energy.

Thus, we probably evolved, as a species, to be efficient energy conservers in order to prevent life-threatening loss of weight. High levels of physical fitness were necessary in order to prevail against the elements, predators and human enemies, and to be able to do the physical labor necessary for survival. With the development of agriculture some ten thousand years ago, the supply of food became somewhat more stable, but hard physical labor was still necessary to assure survival.

While the industrial revolution reduced the number of people involved in farming and put many to work in factories, physical labor was still part of the life of everyone except the wealthy. Most people

---

*A calorie is the amount of heat necessary to raise the temperature of one gram of water one degree Celsius. A large Calorie (also written as kilocalorie—1,000 calories) is the amount of heat needed to raise one *kilogram* of water one degree Celsius. The large Calorie is the one commonly used to describe the energy in food or the energy cost of exercise. Since the large Calorie is now commonly written with a lower-case c, I will follow that practice in this book.

†For a table giving the percentage of the U.S. population deviating from desirable weight, see the Appendix.

did not have a surplus of food, and it was clearly still desirable for them to be energy conservers and to eat foods high in energy density, such as fats and sugars, whenever possible. Wealthy, plump people were viewed with envy. Because the rich lived in cleaner, more healthful conditions than the poor, they were less susceptible to many diseases. They did not have to spend long hours in physical labor, and they had plenty to eat. Our parents and grandparents, especially those who came from countries where life was hard, naturally encouraged us to eat rich foods and hoped that we would be able to lead lives of leisure. Similarly, foods heavy with fats and refined sugar, which had been scarce or unavailable to many of our ancestors, were highly valued, and with improved economic conditions, more people had ready access to these foods.

As technological development accelerated, we became increasingly successful at reducing the energy-consuming demands of work. We acquired labor-saving devices in factories and homes, fewer people worked on farms, and more were engaged in white-collar jobs where they sat at desks all day. The idea that physical exertion was something that you avoided if at all possible was common.

Although many people now accept in theory the idea that exercise is healthful, the lengths they will go to in order to avoid it are ludicrous. It's quite common to see someone waiting several minutes for an elevator to go up or down one flight, instead of using the stairs. Escalators and moving sidewalks abound, while it becomes more and more difficult even to *find* the stairwells in many modern buildings —and they tend to be rather uninviting places, presumably to be used only in case of fire. Then there's the automobile, whose dominance is unquestioned in our society. In fact, many cities and towns make little or no provision for walkers. Two colleagues and I once tried to get to Old San Diego from the center of town on foot. We first realized we might have a problem when our requests for directions were met by puzzled responses. As we went along, we found ourselves looking in vain for sidewalks and even crossing a few highway approaches. We finally got there despite the lack of encouragement, but decided to take the bus back to the hotel.

All the technological developments that reduced the necessity of physical exertion were viewed with great satisfaction by a society whose values were molded during a time when most of us had to work too hard and found it difficult to get enough to eat.

Of course, as we learned to substitute fossil energy for human energy, we also learned to eat somewhat less, lest we blow up and explode altogether. In fact, the average daily intake of calories in the United States has continued to decline in recent years, to about 1,500 for women and 2,400 for men.

The result of all these influences is a population that is far too sedentary for its own good. Surprisingly, the widespread problem of overweight in our society *doesn't* arise from our eating too much; in fact, overweight people generally eat less than thin people. *The problem arises from our abnormally low levels of energy expenditure.*

A recent study of three thousand people, reported in the *British Medical Journal,* showed that those who were fattest tended to eat *least,* while those who were lean generally ate the most. Dr. Jean Mayer, the well-known nutritionist, and his colleagues studied the eating and exercise habits of fat and thin teenage girls and came up with the astonishing finding that, on the average, the fat girls ate considerably less than their thin age-mates. But films of the girls at play revealed the thin girls were far more active than the chubby ones. Clearly the fatness was due to lack of exercise, not to overeating. Of course, chubby people are likely to do poorly in athletics, resulting in avoidance of athletic activities, and the degree of fatness increases even more. Thus a vicious cycle is born.

What happens to most of us is that we gradually accumulate weight between the ages of twenty and fifty. We add one or two pounds a year and one day wake up to find ourselves carrying around twenty to sixty pounds of excess fat. We realize that we don't look good, that we don't feel good, and that this excess fat is likely to shorten our lives. So we resolve to go on a diet, as if our weight gain were the result of overeating. Actually, it's far more likely that it has resulted from a reduction in our daily activity.

When we leave school and join the adult world, most of us take sedentary jobs. We spend our nights in front of the TV. We have less access to sports facilities and less free time. We get into the habit of driving everywhere and of using elevators instead of stairs.

We raise our children to be as inactive as we are. Twenty to thirty years ago, several studies showed that American children were extremely unfit compared to their counterparts in other countries. If the gap has closed at all in recent years, it is because many other countries have become as affluent as we are, and their children, driven everywhere instead of using their feet or a bicycle, are becoming as unfit as American youngsters. And millions of children have substituted TV watching for active play.

The low-energy lifestyle is biologically and psychologically unsound. Along with our increased consumption of refined sugars and fats, and the stressful environment that we find ourselves in today, low energy expenditure has been the critical factor in the increase in overweight and the "lifestyle diseases": heart disease, chronic tension, high blood pressure, adult-onset diabetes, and back disorders. Overweight is merely one of the outward symptoms of what have been called hypokinetic diseases (*hypo-* meaning under, *kinetic* meaning movement), so when we take action against overweight, we will at the same time be fighting these serious health problems.

The surest way to long-term weight control and robust health is to move from a *low-energy* to a *high-energy* lifestyle, along with adopting sensible nutritional habits and effective techniques for the management of stress. A high-energy lifestyle is one in which the amount of calories you take in and the amount you use up are both high. That is, you have a high throughput of energy. You can maintain a given weight by taking in and utilizing a lot of calories, just as you can with a few, but the former is much more psychologically and biologically sound than the latter.

Aha! you say. Now I understand. This is an exercise book. Forget it. I've tried exercise, and it doesn't work for me.

You're both right and wrong. This is in a sense an exercise book. But whereas most such books prescribe one kind of exercise for everyone, this one is going to show you how to increase your level of energy expenditure in the way that's right for *you.*

Maybe you're the type who cringes when the word "exercise" is mentioned, possibly because you were awkward in sports and games as a child, and tended to shy away from physical activity. Or maybe you were active as a child but are now stuck behind a desk all day and "don't have the time" to exercise. Or maybe you've tried a jogging or calisthenics program sometime within the past couple of years and soon gave up, discouraged by the lack of instant success.

If you're any of these people, this book is for you. It will show you how your energy throughput (the rate at which you use up the calories you consume) can be increased naturally, even within the context of a very busy schedule, and without any of the unpleasant consequences sometimes associated with strenuous exercise. A variety of strategies will enable you to increase your activity level gently, gradually, pleasantly, until over a period of months you become a high-energy person who no longer has to worry about weight.

Readers looking for a quick fix for their weight worries won't find it in these pages. Instead, you'll find a scientifically valid analysis of this tremendously widespread problem, showing why people who have adopted high-energy lifestyles have no difficulty controlling their weight despite high caloric intakes which include foods dieters consider taboo. Indeed, one of the ironies of this whole problem is that low-energy people are often on a perpetual diet and feel guilty when eating such things as cake and ice cream, whereas high-energy people usually eat without restraint and with great gusto. One of my patients, for instance, realized that walking three miles more than she normally did on any given day would balance a 300-calorie dish of ice cream. Before this discovery, she was resigned to the idea that she could never again have ice cream, one of her favorite foods, without jeopardizing her fragile caloric balance. By coupling the 300 calories of exercise with the 300 calories of ice cream, she was able to maintain her caloric balance and enjoy her mint chocolate chip much more than ever before.

What happened to me over the course of two years is another good illustration of how a high-energy lifestyle enables you to eat more and weigh less. In my youth, I had been involved in sports all year round, and after college was a physical education teacher and coach for a number of years, taking part in a good deal of physical activity in connection with my job. When I began to specialize in the physiology of exercise and stopped coaching, I exercised a good deal less, though I did continue to play basketball and tennis a few times a week. I began to think I was getting old, because playing basketball at full speed a couple of days in a row left me tired.

This pattern continued until a few years ago, when I began doing preliminary work for this book during a vacation. As it happened, my next-door neighbor was also writing a book. We both found that at about four in the afternoon we felt a great need to leave our desks and do something active, so we began running together. When I went back to work after vacation, I found myself wanting to run on days when I didn't play basketball, and thus began exercising almost every day.

As a result of this increase in physical activity—from about three days a week to six days a week—I probably added something like 15 miles of running to my weekly activity. Using a rule of thumb of about 100 calories per mile, that works out to about 1,500 calories per week. Multiplied by about 40 weeks (taking into account weeks when for some reason I couldn't get in my full quota of exercise), this added up to a yearly weight loss of 17 pounds, or 34 pounds over the two years. As it turned out, I lost about 15 pounds over those two years without trying to—not the 34 pounds I could have been expected to lose if I had maintained my normal diet. Obviously I was eating more than I had before—about 750 calories a week more—and I was weighing less. Of course I really didn't have to do any calculations to realize I was eating more: I had doubled the size of my breakfasts so I could get through my noon-hour exercise without becoming too hungry.

This is precisely the kind of pattern that should be much more common in our society. Of course, my case is a bit extreme, because I was able to increase my exercise by 15 miles a week without much difficulty. But many people can lose weight simply by increasing their routine exercise: exercise that would not be considered a workout. By routine exercise I mean walking to the store instead of driving, taking the stairway instead of the elevator or escalator, and other activities that might be called "walking about." Some of my patients at the weight control center have purchased pedometers to keep track of their daily exercise, and many of them have found that they are able to increase their routine walking from as little as one to as much as seven or eight miles a day without difficulty.

Before we get to why you shouldn't think of dieting as the way to control your weight on a long-term basis, let me say something about this business of taking charge of your own weight and well-being. We are progressively losing control over our lives. Our complex society makes it increasingly necessary to rely on specialists to help us take care of our houses, cars, business affairs, and selves. In the area of health, we have tended to devalue healthful day-to-day living, and to overvalue the ability of specialists to repair damage *after* it is done. But *we have the power to build up our bodies, to prevent damage, by increasing the extent to which we use them.* The degenerative diseases that are now among our main killers and cripplers are actually diseases of *disuse* rather than the result of wear and tear—diseases peculiar to affluent societies such as ours, where we eat the wrong things and use our bodies too little.

As you progress through life, you progress also through a series of medical specialists from pediatricians to gerontologists. Through it all, the only constant is you. Only you can be aware at all times of all those life activities affecting your health. The importance of personal health habits has been clearly shown by Dr. Lester Breslow and his colleagues at the UCLA School of Medicine, who found that life expectancy from age forty-five on is as much as eleven years greater among people who take care of themselves by exercising regularly, getting seven to eight hours of sleep each night, eating three meals per day, maintaining moderate weight, avoiding smoking, and drinking little or no alcohol.

You have the primary responsibility for taking care of yourself— by adopting positive health habits; by insisting that people in the health professions, in addition to treating you when you're sick, help you to stay healthy by teaching you how to take care of yourself; and by being sensitive to the effect that any particular therapy, drug or activity is having on you. In fact, some evidence suggests that taking charge of yourself may be important in the process of losing weight and keeping it off. Most studies of overweight people who have lost weight in therapeutic situations show that the large majority gain all or most of it back. But a recent study by Dr. Stanley Schacter of Columbia University provides data to support my impression that many overweight people *do* lose weight and keep it off for many years. These people don't show up in the statistics because most don't go into therapeutic weight-loss programs. They simply decide one day to take charge of their weight and well-being, find out what to do and do it. Schacter found that of those people interviewed who had a history of obesity and had actively attempted to lose weight, 62.5 percent had succeeded in losing weight (average of 39 pounds for the men and 29 for the women) and keeping it off for many years at the time of the interview (thirteen years for the men and eight for the women). A further 13 percent had lost substantial amounts of weight but were still somewhat overweight. Dr. Schacter didn't report on whether the successful people used diet or exercise, but as we'll see throughout the book, it is quite likely that exercise was a major part of their weight-loss program.

A great many people in our society think that taking care of themselves—getting in shape, as we like to call it—necessarily involves eating less than they do, and so the first step in their get-in-shape program is to go on a diet. Let me explain why this is the *wrong* approach.

2
The Trouble
with Dieting

The claims of some diet books to the contrary, the law of conservation of energy *does* apply to humans: if you take in more calories than you use up, the excess will be deposited as additional weight, and if you take in fewer than you use up, you will lose weight. In short, calories *do* count.

Thus the bottom line of all reducing diets is that you cut down on your calorie intake, although this unpleasant fact is sometimes disguised by the instructions in certain diets to "eat all you want" of certain foods. The monotony of eating a limited variety of foods, however, usually leads to a reduced total caloric intake. How much celery or grapefruit can you eat?

Certainly the fastest way to lose weight (temporarily, at least) is to cut down drastically on your food intake—that is, go on a diet. And there is no shortage of diet books, each with its "revolutionary" new technique for quick (and, of course, effortless) weight loss. Indeed, the very existence of so many different diet books is evidence that there is no one diet formula which really leads to permanent weight control —or everyone would already know about it.

But dieting—as millions of men and women know only too well— is fraught with pitfalls. One very common pattern is as follows: for cosmetic or health reasons, you go on a low-carbohydrate diet and eat a very restricted range of foods. You lose five to ten pounds the first week and three to six pounds the second week. You feel good about the weight loss but lethargic, since without carbohydrates as a fuel, your muscles cannot work effectively. You find it difficult to continue depriving yourself of so many of the good things in life, but though you've already lost a substantial amount of weight, you haven't yet reached your goal, so you apply willpower and remain faithful to the diet.

However, the rate of weight loss diminishes to one or two pounds a week, and you wonder what you did wrong. One week you find that you lose less than a pound, and you're discouraged. You have reached the scourge of dieters, the dreaded plateau.

One night at a friend's house, an especially tasty dessert is served and you can't turn down a small piece. The next day you find you've *gained* a pound, even though the one piece of cake amounted to only a few hundred calories. Oh, the wages of sin! When you mention the decelerating weight loss and the cake episode to friends or your doctor, they smile knowingly. "Come on," they seem to be implying, "where are you stashing the cookies, or are you sleep-walking to the refrigerator at night?"

You decide fate doesn't will you to lose more weight, so you go off the strict diet; but to maintain your new lower weight, you add only a few hundred calories a day to your intake. To your horror, you gain three to five pounds in a week. You conclude that there's something wrong with your metabolism, say to hell with the whole enterprise, and go back to your pre-diet eating pattern. Quickly your weight returns to "normal"—that is, to where it was before you started. Friends look at you pityingly, and you suffer one more blow to your self-esteem; once again, you've failed to achieve self-mastery in an important part of your life.

If you've experienced a pattern like this once or more, you're not alone. *Perhaps as many as 90 percent of people who lose weight by going on diets return to their pre-diet weight within a year or so.*

Why are people able to lose ten or fifteen pounds without much difficulty on any of the dozens of diets that are readily available, only to find that continued loss of weight becomes progressively harder, even though they continue to diet faithfully? And why is it so easy to gain the weight back, even when you seem to be eating less than before you started the diet?

This pattern of repeated weight loss followed by weight gain, which has been called the "rhythm method of girth control," is one of the commonest and most frustrating problems of our time. Recent scientific research has begun to uncover the physiological bases of this problem. Certain changes that occur in the body on a low-calorie diet make it progressively harder to lose weight and keep it off. *It is not simply a question of inadequate willpower.*

For one thing, as we reduce our food intake, we reduce at the same time our intake of all the nutrients in food. Besides the many nutrients scientists have identified as important in preventing various diseases, there are also a number of micronutrients and trace elements in food which play important roles that are not yet fully understood. When you drop your caloric intake to low levels to lose weight or avoid gaining, you may well be getting insufficient amounts of some critical nutrients even if you take vitamin and mineral supplements. The science of nutrition is still in its infancy. How much selenium do we need for optimal health? How much zinc? No one really knows for sure. The pill that contains all the essential nutrients in the right amounts hasn't yet been invented, in spite of the claims made in advertisements.

The large amount of processed food we eat makes this problem of ingesting enough nutrients even more acute, since many essential nutrients are lost in processing. Of course, manufacturers frequently "enrich" the foods, but they can't put back into food nutrients that are still unknown or imperfectly understood.

Then there's all the sugar we consume (24 percent of the average American diet). Since processed foods and sugar provide many calories but few nutrients, we are left with a small amount of food from which to acquire almost all our essential nutrients—and the dieter, who presumably consumes some processed foods as part of his diet, is left with even less. The body probably senses these nutrient deficiencies and cries out for more: this may be the origin of those terrible cravings to eat that attack dieters. People who consistently restrain themselves from eating as much as they want may be fighting a physiological survival mechanism. No wonder they lose the battle more often than they win!

Some fascinating studies of such "restrained eaters"*—perpetual dieters—have shown that when they are placed in experimental situations where the inhibitions to eating are removed, they tend to eat far more than people who don't restrain their eating. In one study, participants were told they were part of an ice-cream-tasting experiment and should eat as much ice cream as they wanted. Before starting to eat, some were told that they would be given something to drink, supposedly in order to clear their palates. They were divided into three groups: one group was given nothing to drink, one was given a milkshake, and the third was given two milkshakes. The people who were not restrained eaters (as determined from a questionnaire) ate less ice cream if they had a milkshake first, and even less if they had two milkshakes. What could be more natural? But the restrained eaters actually ate *more* ice cream following one milkshake than if they did not have one—and the ones who had two milkshakes ate still more!

The restrained eaters seemed to suffer a kind of motivational collapse when the inhibitions to eating were removed by the experimental situation. Subsequent studies showed that when restrained eaters have alcoholic drinks, which presumably *reduce* their inhibitions, they tend to eat more. When they are in anxiety-provoking situations they also eat more, perhaps because habitually restraining themselves from eating is emotionally draining, and it is hard to exercise this control with the added stress of anxiety.

Social pressures affect restrained eaters as well. They are usually able to control themselves when eating with others, but tend to go on eating binges when no one is watching. This characteristic of restrained eaters in certain situations may well be an attempt by the body to make up for chronic deprivation of nutrients, and may be one

---

*Restrained eaters are not necessarily overweight. Some of them can maintain a low weight by eating very little; thus they have a "weight problem" even though they're of average weight.

of the central mechanisms underlying the yo-yo pattern of loss and gain reported by so many people with weight problems.

Needless to say, binge eating is usually accompanied by such guilt that whatever pleasure might be obtained from the food is largely cancelled out. And regaining unwanted weight is terrible for the ego.

If these urges are looked at as signals from the body that some essential nutrients are lacking, then we can see the problem as physiological rather than psychological. We will be less likely to look for some deep-seated psychological basis for overeating. What we *will* do is seek ways to increase the amount of energy we use up, so that we can take in sufficient amounts of food to satisfy our fundamental physiological needs.

Another reason why dieting has such a low success rate has to do with the composition of the tissue lost when dieting. In a fascinating experiment at Washington University, Dr. Lawrence Oscai and colleagues showed that in rats which lost weight through exercise, almost all of the lost tissue was fat and only a small amount was protein, while the rats that lost the same amount of weight through caloric restriction lost *twice* as much in the form of protein. Furthermore, the calorie-restricted rats had much smaller hearts than the exercised rats. Exercise appears to stimulate protein synthesis in the heart and other muscles, thereby preventing much loss of lean tissue, while at the same time taking large amounts of fat from the fat depots of the body.

Studies with overweight women and men have also shown that when weight is lost through dieting alone, more lean tissue is lost than when exercise alone or a combination of exercise and diet are used. For this reason, a person who loses weight through diet alone will appear fatter than someone who loses the same amount of weight through exercise.

Dieting is counterproductive in another way, too. The body's general metabolic rate is partially determined by food intake. When you reduce your caloric intake without increasing your physical activity, the body lowers its general metabolic rate at the same time, as though defending itself against precipitous weight loss—probably an evolutionary survival mechanism that served us well in the past during times of want. And each subsequent time you go on a diet, the metabolic rate drops faster and takes longer to return to normal.

Let's say you go on a 1,000-calorie-a-day diet. With the resulting lowered metabolic rate, your daily caloric *expenditure* will diminish too, and may fall to as little as 1,000 calories, thus balancing your 1,000-calorie intake. Result: no caloric deficit and no weight loss. *By going on a diet, you're actually making it harder for your body to lose fat!*

The Yo-yo Pattern

Recent research suggests that it may actually be healthier to maintain a stable weight at a relatively high level than to repeat the cycle of loss and gain over and over again. Several years ago, Dr. Jules Hirsch and colleagues at Rockefeller University showed that in the early years of an animal's life, fat tissue grows as a result of increases in both the size and the number of individual cells. It was thought that after maturity, any change in the amount of fat tissue is due to changes in *size* of the individual cells, but that no further change in the *number* of cells occurs; and that the total number of fat cells formed in childhood influenced the degree of overweight later on, since the person continues feeling hunger until the cells are "filled up." It was believed that if the development of large numbers of fat cells in childhood and adolescence could be prevented, the tendency to overweight later in life might be controlled.

But more recent studies have suggested that adult animals can have increases in *both* the size and the number of fat cells in their bodies (though the primary increase is in the size)—and that when animals are put on reducing diets, the number of cells does not diminish, even though their size does. Although the weight may be lost, the extra fat cells remain in the body, so after the diet is over the animal will tend to return to a higher stable weight than before. Thus the more times a person goes through this cycle, the more fat cells will be developed and the higher the person's "comfortable" weight will be.

So much for the general disadvantages of going on diets. What about specific different types of diets? What do they do for you (if anything), and more to the point, what do they do *to* you?

Low-Carbohydrate Diets

Low-carbohydrate diets are often used in weight-loss centers. On the surface they seem quite sensible, since the American public has come to think of carbohydrates as fattening—and certainly many of the most calorically dense foods, such as cakes and candies, have many carbohydrates (in the form of sugar) in them. Furthermore, carbohydrates make up such a large portion of most people's diets that by simply eliminating them, you can immediately cut down markedly in calories consumed.

What these diets usually permit is fairly large amounts of protein. The Stillman Diet, for example, allows you to have bacon and eggs and a roll for breakfast, and then all the lean meat, poultry, fish, eggs, and low-fat cheese you want. Sounds pretty good, doesn't it?

The low-carbohydrate diets are also appealing because they usually produce a quick weight loss of five to ten pounds the first week, which encourages the dieter. How does this happen? After all, a ten-pound weight loss corresponds to about 35,000 calories. Since an average person uses about 2,000 calories per day, it seems that it should take at least seventeen days of complete fasting to lose that much weight.

Most of the initial loss is in the form of water. A diet low in carbohydrates will lead to depletion of carbohydrates in the muscles and liver, along with a release of the water stored with the carbohydrate. Presto! A dramatic loss—though of lean body weight, not fat weight. But this water loss is a one-shot deal. The second week's weight loss may be half of the first week's, and by the third or fourth week a loss of one to two pounds per week is usual.

Even this wouldn't be bad if it continued indefinitely. However, what commonly happens is that the rate of weight loss keeps slowing down until one week no weight is lost at all. Then the dieter is apt to believe there's something wrong with his metabolism. To make matters worse, if he eats even a tiny additional amount of food, the body is extremely efficient at storing it, and he may actually gain weight. The discouragement of being unable to continue losing, combined with the stress of dieting, more often than not knocks the person off the diet, and the lost weight quickly returns.

An important disadvantage of low-carbohydrate diets is that carbohydrate is the main fuel for physical activity, so if it is excluded you become fatigued, your exercise capacity is diminished and your ability to use up the calories you eat is reduced.

A particularly unhealthy variant of the low-carbohydrate diet is the Atkins Diet, which allows you to eat all the fats you want. With most low-carbohydrate diets, the body goes into a state called ketosis, in which ketone bodies (acid chemicals) are formed from fats that are incompletely burned. This may cause gout, kidney trouble or liver problems, and odd-smelling breath. But the Atkins Diet, by adding unrestricted intake of fat to its high protein level, encourages not only ketosis (which is magnified because there is no provision for large amounts of liquids to flush out the acids) but also cholesterol buildup and resulting danger to the cardiovascular system. High-fat diets have also been associated with cancers of the colon and breast.

High-Carbohydrate Diets

The *high*-carbohydrate diet is a relatively recent development in the weight-control area. One example is the weight-loss diet of Nathan Pritikin, which includes only 10 percent protein and 10 percent fat in its 600 calories per day, and eliminates coffee, tea, alcohol, and sugar. The bulk of the diet is in the form of complex carbohydrates, mainly vegetables. Because vegetables are so low in caloric density, you can eat a large volume of food on this diet, which helps to provide a feeling of fullness. However, so much fiber can be upsetting to the system, the protein allowance of only 60 calories a day is well below the recommended protein levels, and the severely limited regimen would probably be boring and unsatisfying to most people.

Another high-carbohydrate diet is described in *The Beverly Hills Diet,* a book that soared to the top of the best-seller list in 1981. This diet involves eating large amounts of fruit; in fact, in the first week, you eat *nothing* but fruit.

The commercial success of this book, which is full of scientifically inaccurate statements, illustrates the gullibility of people in search of the magical cure for their weight problems. Drs. Gabe Mirkin and Ronald Shore have pointed out several potential hazards of this diet, including diarrhea, dizziness due to extremely low blood pressure, potassium deficiency, cardiac arrhythmia, hair loss, and extreme weakness.

Undoubtedly, many people have lost weight on this diet, probably because of its requirement that you not eat other types of food at the same time. Restricting variety does lead people to eat less. But most of these people probably regained the weight when they returned to a normal diet.

The Ultimate Diet: Fasting

The most radical reducing regimen is a complete fast. If you have plenty of excess fat, you should be able to provide the necessary energy for life from this storage depot without eating anything at all. Theoretically a person who normally uses up about 2,000 calories per day should be able to lose about seventeen pounds of fat each month on a complete fast (plus another ten to fifteen pounds of water from lean tissue as the body's carbohydrate is depleted). But the weakness that usually accompanies the fast leads to a marked reduction in exercise and thus in the rate of expenditure of calories.

People who fast usually take multivitamins to provide the vitamins, minerals, and trace elements necessary for normal physiological functioning, but in the present state of medical knowledge about the physiological roles of various substances, relying on pills is not the ideal way to obtain all the necessary nutrients. Also, when you fast, a number of minerals and a lot of water are lost. One result is postural hypotension, in which the person has abnormally low blood pressure, leading to dizziness and possible collapse whenever the brain receives insufficient blood, usually when you stand up too quickly. The loss of minerals may upset a number of physiological processes, including some that are as yet unknown.

Another problem of fasting is that lean tissue is lost along with fat. This occurs when the liver converts protein to carbohydrate in order to keep blood sugar from falling. The central nervous system ordinarily requires blood sugar (glucose) for its metabolism. The weakness and shakiness that often accompany fasting are probably due to depletion of the body's carbohydrate stores and reduction in blood glucose.

As with low-carbohydrate diets, ketone bodies are formed and pile up in the blood when you fast. When the brain finds it difficult to obtain sufficient glucose for its metabolism, it can adapt to some extent by using circulating ketones, which still have much of the original energy of the fat bound up in them. When the level of ketones in the body fluids increases this way, ketosis develops. Some researchers who specialize in weight loss have been able to keep their patients in a state of ketosis for several months without any apparent harm. However, the long-term consequences of such an abnormal state are unknown.

Finally, the liver and kidneys are put under considerable strain in handling unusual metabolic and excretory functions, with the possibility of damage if the fast is prolonged.

Considering all the possibly harmful consequences of fasting, it certainly should not be undertaken without careful medical supervision.

Protein-Sparing Modified Fast

In order to mitigate some of the harmful effects of complete fasting, diets that provide small amounts of protein have been formulated. These protein-sparing diets are designed to prevent the loss of lean tissue that occurs with fasting.

Drs. Bruce Bistrian and George Blackburn of Harvard Medical School are perhaps the best-known advocates of the protein-sparing modified fast. Their diet includes a small amount of complex carbohydrates in addition to about 75 grams (300 calories) of protein per day in the form of lean meat. But even these physicians argue that the patients who are most successful at losing weight and keeping it off are those who use the diet as only one part of a multifaceted program of behavior modification, nutrition education, and exercise.

It certainly isn't sensible to rely on liquid formulas when the highest-quality protein is found in regular food. Many dieters prefer a completely prescribed formula so that they don't need to make any decisions—or even face real food at all. In this way they feel they'll avoid temptation. However, this artificial expedient doesn't encourage the permanent behavior change that is essential if weight is to be kept off.

The Balanced Weight Loss Diet: A Temporary Expedient

Radical diets are psychologically and physiologically stressful, and may be harmful as well. They do not help you alter your eating habits in a permanent way, and they don't do anything about our unhealthily low levels of energy expenditure—in fact, they tend to make them even lower. They frequently provide quick weight loss, but in most cases the weight is soon regained. Very high-carbohydrate diets, while more sensible than low-carbohydrate diets, are usually inadequate in protein to maintain lean tissue.

Reducing diets do have their place when you want or need to lose weight more quickly than can be accomplished by increasing your energy expenditure alone, but such a diet shouldn't be a radical departure from the balanced nutrient intake required by the body. I'll describe a sensible temporary reducing diet in chapter 10. But even the best diet is only a temporary expedient.

Diets do nothing to help you *keep* the weight off permanently. A diet is something you go on, and when you go off it, the weight almost always returns because your lifestyle has not changed. The only way to accomplish permanent weight control is to change your lifestyle in a permanent way.

Remember: excess fat is a *symptom* of a low-energy lifestyle. Only by altering the underlying *cause* can you achieve the permanent effect you want. If you act like a trim and fit person, eventually you will become one.

3

Why Exercise Works

"How can exercise make you lose weight? Don't you have to burn up 3,500 calories just to lose one pound of fat?" This is the first of the three most commonly heard objections to the idea that exercise can play a significant role in weight control. Certainly using up the 3,500 calories in a pound of fat takes a lot of exercise—about ten hours of rapid walking, for example, nearly twelve hours of bicycling, or about six and a half hours of racquetball (see the Appendix for the energy-expenditure values of a wide variety of activities).

But nobody needs to or should lose a whole pound at one time. After all, you don't *gain* a whole pound at once.* Fat accumulates slowly, over months and years, as a result of a lifestyle in which a positive energy balance—taking in more calories than you burn—is maintained. The logical and healthful way to get rid of fat is *gradually,* by altering your lifestyle so that you maintain a *negative* energy balance (using up more calories than you take in), and when your weight is where you want it, by maintaining an even balance between calories ingested and used.

---

*The sudden gain you sometimes see after eating a big meal or the loss of several pounds during an exercise session is due mostly to retention or loss of fluid.

For example, by simply increasing your daily energy expenditure by 300 calories for about 300 days out of the year, you can lose (or avoid gaining) over twenty-five pounds per year! 300 calories is the equivalent of about twenty to thirty minutes of running, or of about an hour of rapid walking—the time it might take you to walk to and from work instead of sitting on a bus or in your car.

"You have to exercise strenuously for it to do any good" is common objection number two. Moderate exercise, many people think, has a negligible effect, so they might as well sit still.

Of course, different kinds of exercise use up different amounts of energy in a given time period. A fast game of racquetball for an hour burns up more calories than an hour of gardening; a half hour of running uses more than a half hour of walking. Compare two walkers, one whose rate is a snappy four miles an hour, and another who ambles along at half that speed. Obviously, in one hour the fast walker will use about twice the calories of the slow walker. But if the goal is distance rather than time, the pace doesn't matter. If both walkers decide to cover, say, four miles, and both are about the same weight, *they will use up approximately the same number of calories,* though they will take different amounts of time to do it.

This surprises many people. They think that ten minutes a day of running, or two hours of tennis on the weekend, is better than, say, a couple of hours each day of moderate-paced walking. Not so. What determines how many calories you use up is the amount of force required to move your body weight through a given distance, and you're going to move your body weight a greater distance in two hours a day of even rather slow walking than in ten minutes of running or a once-a-week game of tennis.

Let's say you weigh 190 pounds and have to travel one mile. If you walk that mile instead of riding, you'll use about 100 calories—and you'll use the same 100 calories whether you walk the distance in fifteen minutes or forty minutes. See the Appendix for tables giving the approximate energy expenditure in selected activities for people of different weights, the amount of weight you might expect to lose per week, and the number of weeks needed to lose ten, thirty, or fifty pounds.

In short, exercise doesn't have to be strenuous to be effective!

"But when you exercise, you get hungrier, so you regain the calories you've used up, and maybe more" is the third common objection to the use of exercise for weight control—and on the surface it seems to make sense. Obviously someone engaged in several hours of strenuous manual labor daily has to increase his caloric intake or he'll eventually waste away. But most of us are not going to become lumberjacks who eat 4,000 calories a day, or champion cross-country skiiers who eat 6,000 per day (while remaining very thin). Rather, will the addition of some thirty to sixty minutes of exercise to the daily activities of a sedentary person so stimulate his appetite that food intake increases?

First of all, remember that *expecting* to be hungry can make you eat even if you don't really want to. One of the patients at the Weight Control Center where I am director of physiology joined an aerobic dancing class. "A lot of the people in my class thought they'd be starving after exercising for an hour," she says, "and some of them went home and ate because they thought they were *supposed* to, not because they were really hungry. I quickly realized that I was *thirsty* after class, but never hungry."

A fascinating study conducted by Dr. Jean Mayer and his associates shows that moderate exercise not only does *not* stimulate appetite, but that it actually appears to suppress it somewhat.

The study divided rats into several groups, which were given differing amounts of exercise: none at all, twenty minutes daily, forty minutes daily, and so on up to several hours a day. The animals were allowed to eat as much as they wished, and a careful record of the amount eaten was kept. The researchers observed that the animals who exercised between twenty and sixty minutes a day ate *progressively less* than those who did not exercise at all beyond the normal movements possible in their small cages. Thus moderate exercise—exercise of up to one hour per day or so—either has no effect on or actually *decreases* appetite.

A recent study by Drs. Rosy Woo, John Garrow and Xavier Pi-Sunyer showed what happens to the appetite of overweight women who increase their exercise. Obese women stayed in a hospital ward, where their caloric intake and expenditure could be precisely measured, for about two months. They were told that the purpose was to investigate metabolism, and that they should not necessarily expect weight loss. The women ate as much as they wanted of a regular mixed diet and snacks; the amount they ate was measured without their knowledge. They expended an extra 600 calories a day by walking on a treadmill, quite a substantial amount. Despite this large amount of exercise, *the women did not increase their caloric intake.*

As a result of the exercise, they lost an average of fifteen pounds, almost all of it fat; and the rate of loss did not diminish as the weeks went on, as happens with dieting. Furthermore, they showed substantial drops in blood pressure. This is the clearest evidence to date that exercise does not increase the appetite of overweight people.

Light or moderate exercise of up to an hour or so daily *does* apparently decrease appetite. In humans and rats, exercise causes an increase in the blood and urine of a substance that suppresses appetite. When this substance is injected into a rat, it suppresses its appetite for up to forty-eight hours. (The amount secreted naturally in the body by exercise, however, would not suppress appetite for this long a period.) As exercise level goes up beyond an hour, so does calorie intake—but only enough to maintain weight. People who are accustomed to a great deal of activity—as our forebears were—*must* eat more than inactive people, or they'll get thinner and thinner. Strenuous exercise does suppress appetite temporarily, but it is compensated for by increased caloric consumption one to two days later.

Why do some inactive people tend to eat more than moderately active ones? Dr. Mayer believes that when we are normally active (and a certain amount of physical activity is normal to the human species), our bodies regulate our food intake precisely, in order to keep us lean and fit. In societies where exercise is a part of everyone's daily life, people tend to maintain their weight at stable levels throughout their whole adult lives. But when our activity level falls below the normal range and we become sedentary, our food-intake mechanism becomes disordered. Our bodies no longer know how much food to take in, and as a result, we often eat more than we need. In fact, an extremely sedentary lifestyle may be so abnormal for humans that we overeat as a form of stimulation.

Dr. Walter Bloom of Atlanta studied thirteen housewives, seven of them grossly obese and six weighing a normal amount. A specially

designed watch that ran only when the patient was standing or walking was strapped to the thigh of each. Thus Dr. Bloom was able to
calculate how much time each woman spent standing, lying down and
sitting. He found that the obese women spent only 35 percent of their
time standing up during the day, while the normal-weight women
spent 53 percent of their time in a standing position.

Yet another study, done at Stanford Medical School, showed that
middle-aged men who exercised regularly had the same percentage of
fat in their bodies as men twenty-five years younger, whereas sedentary men generally get fatter as they get older, increasing their percentage of body fat from 15 percent to almost 30 percent between the
ages of twenty and sixty.

Physical activity not only keeps you from gaining weight, but allows you to lose weight even if you don't diet at all. Dr. D. L. Moody
and her associates put eleven overweight college women on an eight-
week walk-jog program. Despite the fact that they didn't change their
diets at all, the women lost an average of twelve pounds of fat each
—and their lean body weight increased by six pounds, resulting in a
net loss of almost six pounds each. And the Stanford Heart Disease
Prevention Program put twenty-two obese women on a seventeen-
week exercise program—two walk-jog sessions and two calisthenics
sessions a week—during which they were told to eat what they
wished. The average weight loss was nine pounds.

How does exercise work to take fat off and keep it off? Let's take
a closer look at the specific factors involved in energy expenditure.

The Basal Metabolic Rate

The basal metabolic rate, or BMR, is the amount of energy you use
up in carrying out the basic physiological processes—that is, the
energy you expend simply by being alive, without any other activity.
The main factor governing your BMR is the amount of lean body
mass you have—all of your weight *not* in the fat tissue, such as
muscle, bone, and body fluids.

This explains why people who have greater muscle development
than others have a higher basal metabolic rate, and why a male and
a female of the same weight will not have equal BMRs. Because

women normally are smaller than men and have a higher percentage of fat in their bodies, they have less lean body mass and a lower metabolic rate. Consequently a woman usually needs to eat a bit less than a man of the same weight. This difference will be discussed in greater detail in Chapter 10.

When you adopt a high-energy lifestyle, you decrease the amount of fat in your body. At the same time, you increase the amount of muscle tissue, and perhaps also the blood volume. Thus, since your lean body mass is greater, your basal metabolic rate increases and you use up more energy in carrying out the basic physiological processes. BMR is measured early in the morning, at least twelve hours after your last meal, to make sure that only your "basal" life processes are functioning. Since this measurement can only be made in a metabolic ward where you're tested before getting out of bed, it is becoming more common to refer to resting metabolic rate (RMR), which can be taken during the morning after resting for a few minutes, as the usual basic level on which other factors are superimposed.

Voluntary Activity

Superimposed on the resting metabolic rate is the energy you use up in all your activities (the EMR, or exercise metabolic rate). If you and your friend are of the same weight, build, and body composition, but you walk more, you'll have a higher level of energy expenditure. If you undertake a jogging, swimming, bicycling, or jazz dancing program, you'll naturally increase your energy expenditure.

Studies have shown that overweight people have a reduced resting metabolic rate per unit of body weight. Lean tissue has a much higher metabolic rate than fat, so that a person with a great deal of fat in his or her body will have a lower RMR *per pound*. But some very obese people may build up an increased amount of lean tissue to support all the extra weight, and some obese-appearing people, such as lifters of heavy weights, may have a great deal of muscle (in a sense, the obese person is continually lifting weight), so that they may have a high *total* resting metabolic rate. Counterbalancing this, however, is the fact that most obese people move around a lot less than lean people, making their total metabolic rate for the day lower than that of lean people.

Furthermore, the metabolic rate *stays* elevated for as long as eight hours after you exercise, so that the amount of calories expended after the exercise can be quite a bit higher than the amount expended before exercising (even if you're inactive both before and after). Why the RMR should remain elevated for so many hours after exercise is not completely understood. One element may be that body temperature increases during exercise, and then gradually, in an hour or more, returns to resting levels. Since the metabolic activity of each cell is speeded up at higher temperatures, some of the post-exercise elevation in metabolic rate is due to the increased temperature.

A second element is the energy "wasted" by the changes in the biochemical structure of carbohydrates and fats that take place as they are transferred into and out of various storage depots in the body. Since aerobic exercise uses up large amounts of carbohydrates, fat, and protein from muscle, liver, and fat depots, after exercise these fuels must be replenished from the diet or from other storage depots. Exercise causes an enhanced turnover of these fuels, leading to a good deal of wasted energy. In other words, a high energy throughput tends to be somewhat wasteful of energy, a type of waste that people interested in weight control will probably find desirable.

A third element, which has only recently been postulated, concerns the energy cost of the synthesis and renewal of cell membranes, enzymes and other cellular proteins. Much more energy is used up in these processes than is ultimately deposited as protein. This is most apparent during periods of rapid growth, when a child eats like the proverbial horse. During exercise, proteins tend to be broken down to provide energy. But this leads to a post-exercise protein synthesis, resulting in a net increase in muscle size after a few weeks of regular training.

Still another possible element in the post-exercise elevation of the metabolic rate has to do with the functions of thyroid hormones, which have been known for some time to increase the metabolic activity of almost all metabolically active cells. It has been discovered that sensitivity to thyroid hormones is markedly increased by exercise, which raises the metabolic rate in most cells and increases lipolysis —the breaking down of fat so it can be transported to the muscles for use as free fatty acids. The more sensitive your fat cells are to thyroid hormones, the more fat you can use up.

Dr. Per Bjorntorp, the eminent Swedish scientist, and his colleagues have suggested that this mechanism "would help to explain the missing energy expenditure that occurs at the beginning of an exercise program, and which cannot be accounted for by the work alone, or by possible changes in the energy intake."

Incidentally, keep in mind that throughout the text and in the tables I have *not subtracted* the caloric cost of simply sitting still from the caloric cost of performing various exercises. However, I have also *not added* to the total calorie cost of exercise the continuing elevation of the metabolic rate *after* exercise and the other thermogenic effects of exercise. I'm assuming, in my estimates of how much exercise you need for specific amounts of weight loss, that these two factors may balance each other out.

Nonshivering Thermogenesis

The third major factor in energy expenditure, which has been the subject of quite a bit of research in the past few years, is nonshivering thermogenesis: the formation of heat in response to eating, cold exposure or stress, but without muscular activity. This mechanism explains why some people who eat more calories than they expend deposit a lot of the excess calories as fat, while others burn them off —why Judy, who regularly eats a three-course dinner, finishes other people's leftovers and is relatively inactive, never gains an ounce, while Fran, her friend of the same age and weight, eats much less than Judy, yet constantly has to watch her weight.

Recent research suggests that nonshivering thermogenesis is markedly reduced with undereating, and increased with overeating. This is probably the basis for the reduction in the metabolic rate which occurs with dieting. The body seems to prevent too rapid weight loss *or gain* by dampening the effects of marked decreases or increases in caloric intake.

Brown Adipose Tissue

It has recently been hypothesized that one place in the body where nonshivering thermogenesis occurs is in brown adipose tissue (BAT) —brown fat. In animals, BAT makes up only 1 to 2 percent of the body weight, but is capable of generating 40 percent of the resting heat production. Unlike ordinary white adipose (fat) tissue, which has a very low metabolic rate, BAT has a tremendously high capacity for increasing its metabolic rate, due to its high concentration of blood vessels and mitochondria (the power plants of human cells), which are responsible for BAT's brown color.

It seems that the BAT turns on—that is, increases in metabolic activity—when the sympathetic nervous system is stimulated. Exercise, eating, cold exposure and stress are all sympathetic stimulators. When we are exposed to cold, we generate heat in order to prevent our body temperature from falling. If this proves inadequate, we start to shiver in order to generate even more heat.

When genetically obese mice, which have very little BAT, are systematically exposed to cold over a period of weeks, their BAT and their capacity for nonshivering thermogenesis increase. Thus the sheltered life most of us lead, in which we are able to avoid most cold exposure, may have contributed to some extent to our weight problems. Perhaps we should make it a habit to expose our bodies to more cold than we customarily do, by turning down the heat to 68 or lower in winter and spending more time outdoors in cold or cool weather.

Several recent studies have shown that exercise in the cold leads to much greater fat loss than the same amount of exercise in moderate temperatures. The subjects in these studies wore warm clothing and were comfortable throughout. The physiological basis for this phenomenon is poorly understood. There may be several different processes involved, including stimulation of BAT. But the implication for overweight people is clear: outdoor winter activity may play an especially potent role in fat control.

Thermogenesis also increases after a heavy meal, apparently to prevent too great a storage of fat. Part of this increased heat production occurs in connection with the digestive process, but some probably takes place in the brown adipose tissue. The thermic effect of a meal seems to be approximately doubled by light exercise after eating. Thus the tradition of a walk after dinner has a sound physiological basis: less of the food you've taken in will be deposited as fat during the hours after eating, and more will be burned off. This is a bonus in addition to the calories used up by the exercise itself.

However, a study by Dr. Karen Segal and me showed that obese women possessed much less of this eating-plus-exercise thermogenesis than lean women. A tendency to lower thermogenesis may predispose certain people to obesity. If you have it, you certainly can become and stay slender, but you may need more exercise and fewer calories to do so than a person without it. I tell my patients that they *may* have a metabolic quirk which makes it harder for them to lose weight and keep it off, so even after they achieve their goal weights they must be especially vigilant. In a sense, they may always have something of a weight problem even if they stay thin.

It is easy to become discouraged if you see yourself exercising as much as someone else, yet not getting the same results. Remember that there is a broad range of normal human variability in thermogenesis, just as in every other area. It's not your fault, and it's not hopeless. The proof is that when a genetically obese strain of mice are put on a treadmill for daily exercise, they invariably grow thin and streamlined. Even if you have a built-in tendency to lower thermogenesis, *you can lose weight and make the loss permanent,* and beating the problem will make you enormously proud of yourself.

Studies in which exercise alone was used as a means of losing weight (subjects were instructed to maintain their normal eating habits), such as those by Moody and the Stanford Heart Disease Prevention Program, mentioned earlier, have found that the amount of weight lost exceeds the amount that could be accounted for by the exercise itself. There are two probable reasons: First, the RMR stays elevated for quite a while after exercising. Second, the repeated stimulation of the sympathetic nervous system through exercise may result in increased amounts of BAT and thus increased metabolic activity. People who exercise a great deal are capable of high degrees of nonshivering thermogenesis when exposed to cold. Maybe the ideal combination is to exercise *lightly* in the cold after eating.*

Although much remains to be discovered in this area, exercise undoubtedly plays an important role in enhancing thermogenesis, and thus in burning up calories at times other than during the exercise itself.

Spot Reduction

"I'm not so interested in losing weight in general. I just want to take off this fat around my buttocks and thighs. Isn't there some exercise that will do this?" Many gadgets are promoted as effortless ways to take inches off your abdomen, buttocks, thighs or upper arms without dieting, in just a few minutes a day of some specific exercise, as if they were going to repeal the law of conservation of energy.

Localized exercise tends to use up fewer calories than total body exercise such as walking, jogging or swimming. This is because localized exercises use smaller muscles, and because these exercises tend to fatigue those small muscles within seconds or minutes. General body exercises, on the other hand, involve large areas of muscle and can be continued for relatively long periods of time.

When done as an adjunct to aerobic exercises, localized exercises *can* improve the strength and firmness of the underlying muscles. This is *not* the same as losing fat, but it will enhance the appearance of your body by reducing flabbiness, which is usually due to a combination of excess fat and poorly toned muscles. So even if little of the fat stored around the exercised muscle is lost, regular exercise of that part of the body will tighten up the area.

Muscle and Fat

In addition to using up excess fat, exercise can indirectly convert fat to muscle. When a muscle is unused, it shrinks and loses some of its protein. Before being used up by the body, the amino acids in this protein generally undergo a chemical change in the liver, which trans-

---

*Note that *strenuous* exercise should be done on an empty stomach, before a meal, while *light* exercise is appropriate after a meal.

forms them into carbohydrates; these are then used by the body, just as are the calories you get from food. If you don't exercise and are taking in more calories than you're using up, the excess will be converted to fat and stored in the body, even as your muscles become smaller.

If you exercise regularly, however, some of the energy used by that exercise comes from the food you take in, and some from the energy already stored in your body—the fat deposits. But the exercise stimulates the synthesis of protein and growth of muscles, so you are increasing protein at the same time as you are losing fat.

Thus when you exercise you're not only getting rid of unwanted fat but are increasing the amount of muscle in your body and thus improving your ratio of muscle to fat. You'll not only look better, but your rate of energy expenditure will increase. Muscle burns up more calories than fat, even at rest. A 160-pound person who is lean and muscular uses more calories in fifteen minutes of sitting still than does someone of the same weight who has a great deal of fat in his body.

This principle is illustrated by a study by Drs. William Zuti and Lawrence Golding, which divided overweight women into three groups. One group reduced calorie intake by 500 calories a day, one reduced intake by 250 calories and increased energy expenditure by 250 calories (resulting in a total deficit of 500 calories) and the third increased expenditure by 500 calories without dieting at all.

As expected, all lost about the same amount of weight (approximately 11 pounds) over the course of sixteen weeks. But the diet-alone group lost less *fat* (about 9 pounds) than the two groups which exercised (about 13 pounds). The exercising groups increased their lean tissue while they were losing weight, whereas the diet-alone group lost about 2½ pounds of lean tissue along with the 9 pounds of fat. (As mentioned earlier, this loss of lean tissue contributes to a reduced resting metabolic rate and makes it easier to gain the weight back.)

Remember that muscle is more dense than fat: that is, a pound of muscle takes up less room than a pound of fat. As you increase your daily exercise, you may find that you look much better to yourself when you stand nude before a mirror, despite the fact that the bathroom scale shows only a small amount of actual weight lost. This is because exercise builds up muscle at the expense of fat. You can therefore lose a lot of inches and dramatically improve your appearance without necessarily losing a lot of pounds. This (and the size of the clothing you can fit into) is just as important as your actual weight in judging your progress.

One of my weight-control patients, a fifty-three-year-old man, finally reached the goal weight he had aimed for. He immediately bought a new wardrobe, only to find that he went on to shrink two more inches around his waist without losing any more weight (he had increased his calorie intake to prevent further weight loss). "You told me I'd probably lose more inches after my weight stabilized," he told me, "but I didn't believe you. Now what do I do with all those clothes?" This was his penalty for working up to five miles of running per day! As you can imagine, he got very little sympathy from my other patients.

In Case You're Still Not Convinced . . .

Exercisers are far more successful in keeping weight off over a long period than non-exercisers. Dr. Jules Hirsch of Rockefeller University recently told me of a not-yet-published study he did with Joel Grinker and other colleagues of a large number of people who had gone to a weight-reducing spa for several weeks. Some months or years later, they were mailed a questionnaire and asked to fill it out. About a third of the people responded; about half of these had either maintained the weight loss achieved at the spa or lost still more weight. The factor distinguishing the successful people from those who had gained back some or all of the weight was that the successful ones had continued to do the exercises learned at the spa. No other factors were related to success in long-term weight control.

Drs. Peter Miller and Karen Sims of Sea Pines Behavioral Institute, Hilton Head Island, got almost identical results when they studied the long-term success of an intensive four-week weight-control program by determining how much the people involved weighed a year after the treatment. Participants were taught various behavior modification techniques, nutritional concepts and the importance of physical activity. Interestingly, the one-year weight losses were not at all related to the weight losses during the program, demonstrating that quick weight loss is not necessarily best for long-term success. When those with the greatest long-term loss (more than 35 pounds lost, with an average loss of 58 pounds) were compared with those who had the least success (less than 20 pounds lost, with an average loss of 7 pounds), the clearest difference between the groups was whether they still engaged in aerobic exercise at least three times a week: 90 percent of the successful and only 21 percent of the unsuccessful did so. The authors of the study conclude that "regular aerobic exercise may be an essential element in long-term weight loss and weight maintenance."

Exercise works even better than behavior therapy. Several recent studies by behavior therapists have evaluated the efficacy of exercise in keeping weight off, as compared to behavioral techniques focused on eating habits. In one study, a dieting-plus-exercise group lost slightly more weight after ten weeks than a group that *just* dieted using behavioral techniques to control eating (an average of 12 pounds versus 10 pounds). But more important, a year later the exercise group had lost an average of more than 16 pounds altogether, while the other group maintained the original weight loss or gained back a few pounds. The behavioral scientists who conducted this experiment, Dr. William G. Johnson and colleagues at the University of Mississippi Medical Center, have refined their clinical program based on their research, and have compared their results with those of other clinics. Their long-term results are considerably better than those of clinics *not* emphasizing exercise as a crucial element in the weight reduction process.

In a study by Drs. Janis L. Peterson of the University of Vermont and Thomas A. Brigham of Washington State University, a group of women using a regular behavioral weight control program with self-control techniques was compared with a group which added structured aerobic exercise to the self-control techniques. Both groups lost about a pound a week, with the exercise group doing slightly better. But during the study, some women in the exercise group exercised only sporadically, and some in the no-exercise group began exercising on their own. When those who exercised (regardless of their group assignment) were compared with those who did not, the exercisers had lost twice as much weight as the nonexercisers, and improved far more in exercise ability and various body measurements (circumference of waist, upper arm and thigh).

In Conclusion . . .

The evidence is rapidly piling up: *exercise is far more effective than diet in controlling weight permanently.* Our bodies were simply not designed for a life of sitting around and eating sparingly. We are clearly meant to consume enough energy to support a good deal of physical activity. Nature never envisioned desk jobs, television, and automobiles when she put the human body together. So let's get going!

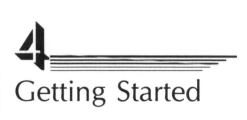

4

Getting Started

Getting started on an exercise program is easier to talk about than to do. For most of us it involves a major change in our ways of thinking and behaving. Willpower is necessary for this change to take place, but it alone is not enough. Research on behavior change has shown that there are two broad steps involved in the process, which can be termed the *why* and the *what*. First, you have to know *why* a particular change is important (for example, why you should exercise regularly). Second, you need to know *what* to do: which specific behaviors to substitute for the old ones.

Almost all behavior is learned, and if it took you a long time to learn the behaviors you have now, you must expect it to take a while to learn new ones. So you must be ready to make a year-long commitment to behavior change. If you can't do that, you may be better off not starting, because without a long-term commitment failure will be likely, and your self-esteem will be damaged.

If a year seems like a long time, keep in mind that diet and exercise programs that promise quick success simply do not work. Think about where you were one year ago. If you had begun to change your behavior then, where would you be today? Given our increasing longevity, you probably have thirty to fifty years or more to live. Isn't it worth a year-long effort to make sure that those years will be healthy and active ones?

In earlier chapters, I've tried to show you *why* you should move from a sedentary lifestyle to a high-energy one. In this and the next two chapters, I'll talk about the *what*. Keep in mind, though, that the suggestions I offer are just suggestions. No one exercise program is right for everyone. Not only are the needs of a sixty-year-old cardiac patient and a chubby twelve-year-old girl quite different, but the needs of any two sixty-year-old cardiac patients will be different. Even when the needs of two people are similar, a particular exercise or dietary regime will affect each differently. In fact, in many studies of the effects of exercise, some subjects do not improve at all while others improve much more than expected, showing that the exercise was far from being equally effective for everybody. So use the information in these chapters to create your *own* exercise program. If you are not getting the results you want, then switch to something else. Many people try a type of exercise or an exercise program that has worked for someone else, and when the pleasurable feelings or health benefits they expect aren't forthcoming, they give up the whole idea. "Exercise? Oh, I tried it, but it didn't work for me."

Listen to your body. It can guide you through the whole process of moving into a high-energy lifestyle. Ignoring the information your body gives you will certainly reduce the effectiveness of the exercise, and may even lead to permanent damage. For example, if you start a jogging program and find that after about twenty minutes of jogging your right knee begins to hurt, stop or slow down. When the knee feels better, gradually resume your former running pattern. But if you ignore this information and continue running, you may damage the knee so much that you can't jog for several weeks or months. Besides, you'll be likely to favor that side while jogging, with the resulting inefficient movement causing damage somewhere else, perhaps in the left hip. Now you've got double trouble!

Your body can also tell you about the amount of strain a given exercise is imposing on you, and how to space your activity throughout the week. It can tell you whether you feel pleasantly exhilarated or just plain worn out after you exercise, and how quickly to progress. Even though exercise physiology has made great strides in determining which exercises are most effective for which purposes, much is still unknown about why certain people respond differently from others. If your body doesn't seem to respond the way you expect it to when you try a certain exercise technique, don't assume there is something wrong with you; there may be something wrong with the technique as it applies to you.

A Program for Behavior Change

When you start an exercise program, you want to give yourself the best possible chance of success. The following steps will do just that:

1. *Assess your own needs* by comparing what you are with what you want to be. For example, are you an eighteen-year-old who doesn't look as good in a swimsuit as you would like to? Are you a forty-year-old with middle-aged spread? Do you find yourself so tense when you get home from work that you need two martinis to relax? Would you like to be 30 pounds lighter? Stronger? Less tense? More energetic? These are the kinds of questions you should ask yourself.

2. *Plan carefully.* If you start haphazardly, you may injure yourself or find that you feel uncomfortable and that your exercise isn't giving you pleasure—with the result that you're less likely to continue or to start any other activity. Study your schedule and find time slots that can be used for exercise: early morning, part of your lunch hour, coffee breaks, the time you spend going to and from work, the half hour before dinner, and so forth.

3. *Start slowly and gradually.* Don't do anything radical at first. Set small, short-range goals that can be attained easily, such as:

* This week I will walk thirty minutes before lunch at least three times.
* At least three times this week I'll go out for a walk during my coffee break instead of having anything to eat or drink.
* This week I'll join an aerobic dance class.
* This week I'll walk five miles more than I walked last week.

Achieving such modest goals will bring you an increased feeling of self-confidence and self-mastery, as well as some modest but clear-cut physiological changes that will make it physically a little easier to attain your next goal.

When I work with overweight patients, I'm constantly urging them to lower their sights. They have a natural tendency to be enthusiastic, and they may think I'll be pleased if they announce ambitious goals for the week. But setting an overly ambitious goal may be an unconscious way of setting yourself up for failure: it's easy to excuse yourself for failing at a difficult task. If you are really serious about changing your lifestyle, you'll set easy goals, achieve them, and move on to more challenging ones gradually. That way you'll have no excuses. You can do it!

4. *Don't push yourself.* If you join a dance or yoga class and find yourself getting extremely tired halfway through, don't force yourself to continue. Just because some exercise is good, more is not necessarily better. Exercise that is inappropriate for you or for the enviromental conditions you find yourself in can be dangerous to health and life. Besides, many people have been turned off exercise altogether by the sore muscles and feelings of debilitation that result from trying to do too much too soon. Pay attention to your body, and quit or slow down when your body tells you to, instead of trying to achieve such external goals as a specific number of aerobic points or a particularly twisted yoga position. One of the surest ways to damage yourself is by trying to gain back in two weeks something you lost over two or twenty years.

5. *Arrange your environment to facilitate goal achievement.* Identify the chains of actions that will result in the desired behavior, and make it as easy for yourself as possible to follow through. For example, if you plan a thirty-minute walk before breakfast tomorrow, go to bed thirty minutes earlier tonight and set the alarm. Make an appointment to exercise with someone else. Buy proper clothing in advance.

One of my patients was a divorced woman with two young children. As a working mother and the head of a single-parent family, she had trouble figuring out how to fit in the exercise I was advocating. I suggested she have her babysitter come fifteen minutes earlier in the morning so she could walk around the block for fifteen minutes before going to work. She also asked the sitter to stay an extra fifteen minutes in the afternoon so she could be dropped off several blocks from her home and walk the rest of the way. And she convinced some of her co-workers to join her in walks during coffee and lunch breaks.

6. *Be flexible.* If you find your first approach to exercise to be disagreeable or ineffective, try a different one. You won't maintain any long-term change in behavior if you find the behavior unpleasant. If you don't like jogging, try walking. If swimming isn't your cup of tea, try bicycling. There are enough choices available to ensure that you'll find something you enjoy.

Similarly, if you've decided to get up and run every morning before breakfast and you find that you can't sleep because you're dreading that early morning ringing of the alarm, try running before dinner instead. If you've been doing an hour of stationary bicycling before bed and then you're too stimulated to relax, try doing it while watching *Good Morning America* or the *Today* show.

7. *Monitor yourself.* Record your activities for a week or two before starting your exercise program, so you'll have a clear base line against which to measure your progress. Then jot down what you accomplish each week in a log or diary: what exercise (including routine walking, stair climbing, raking the leaves, etc.) you do each day, for how long, where and with whom, the surroundings, and your feelings. Looking back over the record of your progress will be deeply satisfying.

You might buy a pedometer to record the distance you walk each week. A pedometer can be worn unobtrusively, but you may want to let it show: it announces that you are serious about becoming a high-energy person. Although pedometers are not very accurate in giving exact mileage, due to variability in stride length, they can tell you how much you've done this week compared to last week, and so on.

8. *Make sure that the new behaviors you're trying to learn are associated with pleasant sensations.* You want to show yourself that it's in your power to provide yourself with pleasurable bodily sensations, which is just another way of saying that it's within your power to make yourself happy. If you undertake a walking, running or bicycling program, for example, start on a beautiful day. Try to do it in beautiful surroundings and, if possible, with someone you like. Do whatever is necessary to make it an enjoyable event. Then, when you think about taking another walk or run, the pleasant aura of the occasion will come to mind, and you'll want to repeat it. When people in a heart disease control program were asked about the factors that

led them to *stay* with exercise over a long period of time, they reported that it was the pleasurable bodily sensations and social interaction that kept them walking, running, swimming, dancing or whatever.

Some people insist that "if there's no pain there's no gain": if it doesn't hurt it can't be good for you. I couldn't disagree more. True, the more you stimulate your system, the more training effect you get, up to a point. But beyond that point, the discomfort that results may actually interfere with the training effect. And if it's unpleasant for you to exercise, you're simply less likely to do it. So start very slowly, progress just to the point of discomfort, and then slow down or stop.

9. *Reward yourself* for successfully completing an exercise session or meeting your exercise goals for the day with a long hot shower or a relaxing bath. For meeting longer-range goals, periodically treat yourself to a massage or a facial, or buy an attractive warmup suit, a new leotard or swimsuit to enhance your self-image.

Some of my patients put a quarter or dollar into a jar after each workout or when they've achieved a weekly goal. When enough money accumulates, they use it to buy themselves something special —often a garment of a smaller size than they've been wearing. Besides giving yourself a present, you'll find it satisfying each time you put money in the jar, because it means a small goal accomplished.

10. *Think pleasant thoughts* during your exercise to reinforce the activity. For example, imagine yourself as you would like to be: looking trim and fit in a bathing suit, or running along easily on a beautiful country road. Or remember the wonderfully relaxed and satisfied feeling you usually get after a workout. Associating this good feeling with the beginning of your exercise will motivate you to continue; and later, you'll be pleased with yourself for having done it instead of giving in to the urge to curl up in an easy chair with a drink or a cup of coffee.

Routine Exercise

The most sensible and easiest way to begin to change your lifestyle is through increasing your routine walking. It's easier than you think to find time to do this, even if you have a full-time job. Here are some possible ways; you can no doubt think of others:

1. Walk to any reasonable destination in your neighborhood, such as the movies, shopping areas or friends' houses. One of my patients made a little map showing the distances from her house to many locations in her town; she found it very motivating to know how far she walked each time. When she first undertook her walking program, friends driving by would constantly offer her lifts, which she turned down pleasantly but firmly. After a while they would just wave, but as time went on, some joined her.

2. If you must drive to a shopping mall (or if you're going to a supermarket to do your weekly food shopping), take a brisk walk from one end of the mall or parking lot to the other before shopping.

3. Get into the habit of parking your car several blocks from your destination.

4. Walk to the next bus stop instead of to the one nearest you; get off a stop or two before your destination.

5. On your lunch hour, walk to a restaurant that is several blocks away.

6. If you usually watch television at night, look at the listings early in the evening, find a half hour or more when nothing special is on, and plan a walk. Walking with a spouse or friend increases the pleasure.

7. Instead of routinely taking elevators and escalators to go up one or two flights, take the stairs. If you have to go up many flights, get off a couple of floors before your destination and walk the rest of the way.

8. Set your alarm clock fifteen minutes earlier than usual and walk to work instead of driving; or park a fifteen-minute walk away from your job.

9. On your coffee break, get out for a brisk ten-minute walk instead of eating. The air and sunshine will be good for you, too. Many people spend all day indoors and hardly ever see the sun. During the winter, make the extra effort to bundle up and get outdoors during your lunch or coffee break. Exercising in the cold leads to

much more fat loss than the same amount of exercise in warmer weather. Consider the winter an opportunity for increased fat loss.

Weight Loss with Routine Exercise

Start with about fifteen minutes of walking a day, at a very relaxed pace of about 2 miles per hour. If you have no lingering fatigue or soreness, increase your walking to a half hour per day, then to forty-five minutes, and finally to an hour. You can do it all at once or break it up into shorter segments (longer periods of exercise are better for cardiovascular fitness, but some evidence suggests that exercising even five minutes at a time provides some training effect). If you also increase your speed to 3 miles an hour, which is a steady but comfortable pace for most people, you'll cover about ¾ of a mile in 15 minutes (get a pedometer to check your distance), and use up about 300 calories in an hour. If you don't increase or decrease your food intake, you'll use some 9,000 extra calories in a month, and lose about 2.6 pounds.*

You can substitute other activities for some of the walking—stair-climbing, for instance. If you weigh 190 pounds, stair-climbing at the rate of two steps per second uses 17.5 calories per minute (going downstairs uses 6.7). If you're overweight or out of shape, don't attempt more than two flights at a time to start with, as this is a very strenuous activity. Two minutes a day of walking upstairs and two minutes of walking downstairs adds up to a yearly loss of 5 pounds, to add to your weight loss from walking and other exercise.

Gradually increase your walking pace. After a month of walking at 3 miles per hour, increase it to 3.5. You'll expend 10,710 extra calories and lose 3 pounds in a month. After a few weeks, increase your pace again, to 4 miles an hour, which is a very brisk pace. This will use 12,240 extra calories a month, for a weight loss of about 3.5 pounds. When you reach 4 miles an hour, you're no longer just doing routine exercise—you're getting an aerobic workout. Routine and aerobic exercise are a continuum rather than two entirely separate activities.

---

*These figures are for a 190-pound person. See the table on page 46 for other weights.

Pounds Lost per Month as a Result of Walking One Hour per Day

Weight	2 mph	3 mph	4 mph
110	1.2	1.7	2.1
130	1.3	2.0	2.4
150	1.4	2.2	2.8
170	1.6	2.4	3.2
190	1.7	2.6	3.5
210	1.9	2.8	3.9
230	2.0	3.0	4.2

Better and Better

As you progress, you'll see an accelerating weight loss, unlike the situation in dieting, where weight loss almost always decelerates as time goes on. Sometimes you may not see the effect of the exercise in the first few weeks, because regular exercise increases muscle and liver glycogen stores, especially in an inactive person who had low glycogen stores to start with. The extra water stored with the glycogen (in lean tissue) may temporarily keep you from losing *weight,* though you are losing *fat* while increasing lean tissue. Since fat is more bulky than lean tissue, there will be a loss of inches and an increased resting metabolic rate—making true weight (fat) control easier in the long run.

Your total weight loss after a year, if you simply walk an hour a day at an average of 3 miles per hour, without changing your eating habits, will be about 30 pounds. If you progress to a full-scale aerobic program, as described in Chapter 6, the potential weight loss is even greater.

If you can progress from walking to running, your potential for using up a lot of calories in a given amount of time increases substantially. For example, let's look at what happens if you add 30 minutes of running, at a 10-minute-per-mile pace (6 miles an hour), to your daily schedule. If you weigh 150 pounds at the beginning of the year, you would use up approximately 11.75 calories per minute, or 352.5 calories in the 30 minutes. If you do this 300 days of the year (I'll allow you some time off for good behavior), it comes to a weight loss of about 30 pounds for the year. If you start at a weight of 200 pounds, you use about 15.2 calories per minute, 456 per session, for a weight loss of about 39 pounds for the 300 days.

Rely on what feels comfortable to you when deciding how quickly to progress. Use the guidelines in the next chapter for heart rate, breathing, and rate of perceived exertion. If walking an hour a day at 3 miles an hour seems quite easy, you can increase your rate without waiting a month. If you're puffing after this much exertion, even when the hour is broken up into ten- or fifteen-minute segments, continue at the same rate until you feel comfortable, and then increase it. Exertion should be *pleasurably tiring:* if it's just pleasurable, you're doing too little; if it's just tiring, you're doing too much.

When you've lost as much weight as you want to, you can increase your caloric intake, provided you continue exercising. For example, if you're using up 400 extra calories a day, you can eat an additional 400 calories. You'll be eating more than you were before—and weighing less.

The table on page 173 in the Appendix shows some additional foods you can eat without gaining weight if you do certain kinds of exercise, and other tables contain the calorie cost of and expected weight loss from many types of exercise. Dr. Frank Konishi has compiled an extensive list of food-exercise equivalents in his book, *Eat Anything Exercise Diet.*

If you don't see a slow, steady weight loss with this program, scrutinize your eating. Are you *expecting* to be hungrier and therefore eating more? Are you telling yourself that since you're exercising now, you can afford to indulge your taste for sweets just a little? *Don't assume you can eat more right away.* You have to *earn* the right to add those calories. If you want to make sure that you don't add to your food intake until you've exercised down to your desired weight, you can either count calories, not going over the amount you normally take in, or substitute complex carbohydrates for some of the meat and fat in your diet (we'll talk more about this in Chapter 9). Because complex carbohydrates are bulky, you'll have the same feeling of satiety, but you'll be ingesting fewer calories (which will speed up your rate of weight loss).

A Note of Caution

Many overweight people start weight-loss programs, usually involving dieting, and the first time they suffer a loss of resolve and eat more than they should, they give up altogether. We have seen that there are physiological and psychological problems with long-term dieting, and that exercise is a better approach. But many people also start exercise programs enthusiastically and for one reason or another (injuries or illness, for example) have to miss a few days or even weeks, leading them to give up this approach also. Taking the long view can reduce the discouragement that results from an interruption of your exercise program. Rather than comparing one day or one week to another, think about whether you did more exercise this *year* than last year. This will show you that you *have* made progress, and may help you resume the program. Think of the gap as a temporary setback within the context of long-term progress, rather than as evidence of inadequate willpower or resolve.

5

Understanding Physical Fitness

Health is a continuum ranging from a state of extreme physical and psychological well-being down to severe debilitation and sickness. I use the term "dynamic health" throughout this book to emphasize that at the upper end of the health continuum, where your organs and psyche are functioning optimally, you are capable of performing at a high level. Your state of health and vitality is expressed in *dynamic* ways rather than by noting the absence of a disease of some sort. That's why we measure dynamic health by how your body performs rather than by the medical tests commonly used to assess lower levels of health.

Dynamic health is a multi-factorial concept, and the elements comprising it are illustrated in the figure on the next page. Though some of the elements are related to one another, each makes a unique contribution to the whole. Since there is no *one* test that can measure the totality of dynamic health, and no *one* type of exercise that can develop all the elements, each component will be examined individually and its relationship to the others explained. (Tension control will be included in Chapter 7, where the ways in which exercise aids in the prevention and treatment of various health problems are discussed.)

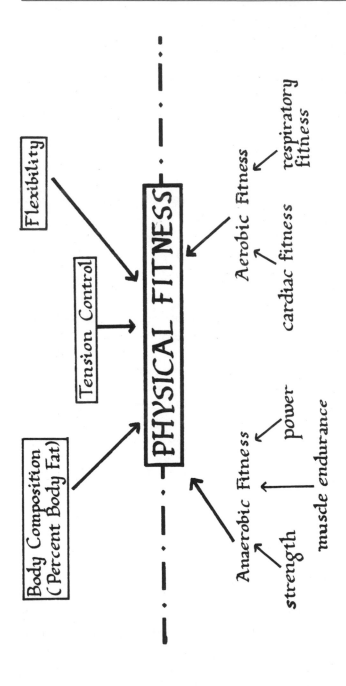

Components of Physical Fitness

Anaerobic and Aerobic Fitness

First is a series of factors that are measured in terms of work performed, and which collectively make up your *physical working capacity*. These are shown below the dashed line in the figure opposite.
These factors are of interest not only because they indicate how
effectively you can perform work but also because they tell about the
health of the organs and systems involved.

Your ability to perform work depends on the extent to which your
muscles can take energy stored in the food you eat and transform it
into mechanical energy, which is what makes the muscles contract
and the limbs move. Two main types of energy release in the body
underlie your physical working capacity: *anaerobic* and *aerobic*.

Anaerobic energy release involves chemical processes in the muscles that release energy without using oxygen. Because these processes
release energy very quickly, they are important in situations where
you want to do a lot of work in a hurry, within a few seconds or a
minute or two—rushing out of a burning house, for instance, or lifting
a heavy piece of furniture. Sports activities such as sprinting, weight
lifting, or leaping in ballet depend on *anaerobic fitness*.

Anaerobic fitness can be subdivided into *strength* (the amount of
force you put into one all-out muscular contraction), *muscular endurance* (the number of contractions that can be completed in a minute
or two), and *power* (the speed with which you can perform work
lasting up to ten seconds or so). All of these are closely related, and
all are dependent on anaerobic energy relase. The types of exercise
that develop anaerobic fitness will improve strength and therefore
carry over to power and muscular endurance as well.

Although anaerobic processes allow you to release energy quickly
—that is, they are high in *power*—you can't continue at that high rate
for more than a minute or so without becoming extremely fatigued,
because anaerobic processes are low in *capacity*. If you want to continue for several minutes or more, you must slow down and allow
aerobic energy release processes to take over.

Aerobic fitness depends on your ability to breathe oxygen into your
lungs, send it into the blood, pump it around the body through the

action of the heart, and use it in the muscles. Although this process is more complex and cannot release energy as quickly as anaerobic processes, it can continue indefinitely.

The activities appropriate for your new high-energy lifestyle are largely aerobic in nature—walking, jogging, swimming, cycling, dancing and so on. There are two reasons for this. First, if you keep the intensity or speed of the activity at a low enough level so that you can continue pleasurably for at least ten minutes and up to an hour or more, you'll use up more calories than if you go all out for one minute. Second, aerobic activities are more effective than anaerobic at stimulating and developing the fitness of the physiological systems basic to lifelong health, such as the circulatory, respiratory, nervous, endocrine and temperature-regulating systems.

The general idea is to work at an intensity of exercise sufficient to stimulate all these systems, but not so high as to require much anaerobic energy release. The reason is that one metabolic end product of anaerobic metabolism is lactic acid, which builds up in the muscle and body fluids to a point where it causes discomfort and pain. Lactic acid also interferes with muscular contraction and relaxation. When you do situps as fast as you can until you reach a point where your muscles hurt and you can't do another situp, it's because lactic acid has built up in the muscles and is interfering with the processes of contraction.

Remember that anaerobic and aerobic fitness are quite independent of each other, so the activities that stimulate and develop anaerobic processes will not develop aerobic fitness, and vice versa. To develop both, you must build both types of exercise into your fitness program.

Assessing Your Anaerobic Fitness

Most of us are interested in knowing how we stack up compared to other people of our sex and approximate age, and such information is helpful in showing us which components of fitness to emphasize in an exercise program. However, keep in mind that your performance on any test is limited to a large extent by anatomical and physiological factors that are part of your hereditary makeup. Because your natural endowment is so critical in determining your test scores, you may find that you score rather well on a particular test, even though you haven't trained for that aspect of fitness. Or you may score poorly on a fitness component you've been working on for a long time. But although heredity is important, it's not the only factor. You can influence your fitness considerably by appropriate exercise and diet. Therefore, view your score as an indication of how you stack up against yourself at another time in your life.

The norm charts, which are based on the performance of a large cross section of people, tell about *average* performance, not necessarily *optimal* performance. Certainly the average level of both aerobic and anaerobic fitness in our society today is too low for optimal health, and almost anyone can eventually become much more fit than the average person.

Also, the average values usually get much worse as the population on which the norms are based grows older. This is simply a reflection of the fact that most people in our society become progressively less fit as they age, not so much because aging per se diminishes their capacities, but as a result of sedentary living and disuse of their bodies. People who maintain an active lifestyle lose their fitness at a much slower rate than the average sedentary person.

So use the assessment procedures to chart your own progress, or to assure that you are maintaining the fitness level you want, and use the norms to provide a rough guide to how you stack up against the general population.

Anaerobic fitness may be measured easily by noting the number of repetitions of certain calisthenics you can complete in a short period of time—say, one minute. The number of situps you can complete in one minute is a good measure of abdominal anaerobic fitness. The test is done with the knees bent at about a 90-degree angle so the soles are flat on the floor. Your ankles should be held down by someone or something, and your hands should remain clasped behind your head throughout. Resting in a lying position is allowed if you cannot keep moving continuously. Norms are shown in the table on page 54.

As your abdominal muscles get stronger, you'll be able to do more situps. Since strong abdominal muscles provide protection against back injury, the anaerobic fitness of this part of the body is important for lifelong health and should be part of every fitness program. In fact,

Norms for One-Minute Situps

	Women	Men
Excellent	35	40
Average	24	30
Poor	14	20

from the point of view of lifelong health, this is the *only* part of the body in which a high level of anaerobic fitness is especially important.

By adjusting the mechanical arrangements in various calisthenic exercises, it's possible to place a fairly high load on the muscles involved. In fact, for most adults who exercise to promote lifelong health rather than to improve sports performance, calisthenics can provide sufficient anaerobic fitness.* Some degree of overall anaerobic fitness is desirable to maintain the tone and firmness of the body. Much of the flabbiness we see in unfit people is due to poor muscle tone in addition to excess fat. In order to obtain a good training effect, you should keep doing the exercise until you feel it hard to do any more. In other words, continue to the point of momentary muscular failure in order to be sure you're stimulating the anaerobic capacity of that muscle.

What Anaerobic Fitness Does for You

Various measurable changes take place in the body as you develop higher levels of anaerobic fitness. You'll see an increase in the size, definition and firmness of your muscles. The connective tissue in your muscles and joints will also become stronger, thereby protecting you from injuries. Within the trained muscles, the metabolic processes and enzymes that subserve anaerobic activities will be enhanced. Thus, you'll be able to release energy anaerobically at a faster rate and for a longer period of time, and will be able to tolerate higher levels of lactic acid before reaching fatigue. The bottom line is that you'll feel strong and will be able to jump higher, run faster, lift heavier objects and perform better in sports that depend on anaerobic fitness.

---

*Specific calisthenic exercises are described in a number of books, including one I helped edit, *Physical Fitness* (Holt, Rinehart & Winston, 1980), and *Jane Fonda's Workout Book* (Simon and Schuster, 1981).

Aerobic Fitness

Any tasks carried on for more than two minutes or so are dependent on aerobic energy-releasing processes and therefore on aerobic fitness. Keep in mind that an activity performed at high intensity for one minute, in which almost all the energy is released anaerobically, is usually followed by a rest interval or a period of easy exercise in which aerobic processes are used to partially oxidize the lactic acid produced during the exercise. If the high-intensity exercise is repeated many times during a game or practice session, the whole session may stress both anaerobic and aerobic processes.

A physiological factor basic to aerobic fitness is *maximal oxygen consumption*, the maximum amount of oxygen a person can utilize per unit of time. This determines the maximal rate at which energy can be liberated through aerobic pathways, so it's central to aerobic fitness.

Let's look at what happens inside your body as you run for four to fifteen minutes or so. Some energy is being liberated anaerobically, but most is released aerobically. Remember that anaerobic metabolism leads to the formation of lactic acid, which interferes with the contraction of the muscle and leads to cramping and pain. Much of the lactic acid is buffered in the body fluids to keep the body from becoming too acid. The buffering process results in the formation of carbon dioxide, a powerful stimulant to respiration. As a result, you feel a need to breathe deeply and quickly, and labored breathing is one of the clearest subjective signs of approaching fatigue: you feel unable to catch your breath. You must slow down because your aerobic processes cannot keep up with the demands of the exercise.

The higher your maximal oxygen consumption, the less use you'll make of anaerobic pathways, and the longer and harder you'll be able to continue exercising before the lactic acid and associated physiological changes cause you to slow down or stop.

In order to have a high maximal oxygen consumption, the organs and physiological systems that take in, transport and utilize oxygen must be operating effectively. For this reason, maximal oxygen consumption is considered by physicians and physiologists as an excellent index of circulo-respiratory health, as well as of aerobic fitness. Even if you're not particularly interested in enhancing your ability to run long distances, you should still be interested in your maximal oxygen consumption for what it tells you about the health of your heart, lungs, circulation, and metabolic function.

Although maximal oxygen consumption is central to aerobic fitness, some recent experiments have suggested that some other physiological measures are also important. One measure we've found extremely useful is the *anaerobic threshold*—that intensity of work above which some of the energy is liberated anaerobically. As mentioned earlier, when you work at very high intensities, almost all of the energy is liberated through anaerobic processes, but when you work at low intensities, as in slow walking, just about all the energy is liberated *aerobically.* If you walked and ran on a treadmill at progressively increasing speeds, you would at first be liberating all the energy aerobically. As the speed reached a level that elicited 40 to 75 percent of your maximal oxygen consumption, you'd begin to liberate some of the energy anaerobically, and if the speed continued to increase, a progressively larger proportion of the total energy released would come through anaerobic metabolism, with a resulting lactic acid accumulation in the muscles and body fluids. Earlier, it was noted that this leads to difficulty in muscular contraction and labored breathing, which in turn signal impending fatigue.

If you were to walk or run steadily at a pace just below your anaerobic threshold, you would feel comfortable and be able to continue for perhaps an hour or two, with fatigue finally occurring for physiological reasons to be discussed later. However, if the pace were somewhat above your anaerobic threshold, lactic acid would be formed and you would probably feel tired within fifteen to thirty minutes. Of course, the further above your anaerobic threshold you work, the faster the lactic acid accumulates and the sooner fatigue occurs.

While you'd probably find it uncomfortable to work at an intensity over your anaerobic threshold, you could do so for a while if you could stand the discomfort, and athletes commonly do so in training and competing. When starting an aerobic program it's sensible to stay at a relatively comfortable level around your anaerobic threshold.

A third factor that may be important in performance of aerobic endurance tasks is the *amount of fat* carried around during the task. Since fat doesn't contribute to the performance of the task, it is merely excess baggage on which energy is squandered when it is moved around. This is why a fat person often has so much difficulty exercising. Even if his circulo-respiratory system is functioning fairly well, exercise can be difficult and discouraging. But as weight is lost and circulo-respiratory fitness is enhanced, a positive cycle develops and the whole process becomes easier.

A fourth important factor in aerobic exercise that is carried on for an hour or more is the *depletion of glycogen from muscles*. Since much of the energy used in exercise comes from glycogen, and since the body doesn't store large amounts of it (in contrast to the amounts of fat it stores), glycogen can reach very low levels in prolonged exercise. Eating a diet with sufficient carbohydrates is the key to maintaining glycogen levels. Thus, people who go on a low-carbohydrate reducing diet frequently find themselves getting tired quickly. The ironic result is that they then reduce their activity, which slows down or stops their weight loss.

The final factor that's important in prolonged exercise, expecially in warm weather, is the *buildup of heat in the body* as a by-product of exercise metabolism. We'll talk about this at greater length on page 78.

Assessing Aerobic Fitness

Aerobic exercises are extremely important for two reasons. First, many sports are carried on for continuous periods of fifteen to thirty minutes or more. Your performance can therefore be influenced by your aerobic fitness (or lack of it, when the power and accuracy you exhibited early in the game suddenly disappear). Further, your chances of being injured increase late in the game when fatigue interferes with your ability to protect yourself at a critical moment. Second, aerobic exercises enhance the functional capacity and dynamic health of the heart, lungs, blood vessels, and the aerobic metabolic pathways in the muscles.

Aerobic fitness may be assessed by measuring the time you require

Norms for the 1.5-Mile Run (minutes)

	Women	Men
Excellent	11	10
Average	14	13
Poor	17	16

for a 1-to-2-mile run or the distance you cover in 12 minutes, as suggested by Dr. Kenneth Cooper of the Aerobics Center in Dallas. The 1.5-mile run is an excellent test, and norms are given in the table above.

But before you go out and do a fast 1.5 miles to measure your aerobic fitness, consider what type of stress this provides. If you've been sedentary for several months or years, you'll probably find the test debilitating and perhaps downright dangerous.

When I first started teaching conditioning courses designed for non-fit college students, I decided to give the students an all-out test on the first day of class so that we could see how they progressed during the term. So I organized a circuit-training program in which the students did a series of calisthenics, weight training, and bench stepping exercises designed to stress all the energy systems and major muscle groups of the body. The circuit was designed to be completed in ten to fifteen minutes. I wasn't surprised to see that some students took longer than fifteen minutes to complete the circuit and that all of them were perceptibly dragging at the end. But I was astonished to see how sad a group they were at the next class meeting two days later! Most of them hadn't yet recovered from the exhaustion caused by the test: they were sore and discouraged, and probably some of them came down with colds due to the extreme stress of the test.

Fortunately, there is a way to assess aerobic fitness without conducting an exhausting all-out test. It involves the measurement of heart-rate response to a standard bout of exercise. A person who is well-trained for aerobic exercise can provide the oxygen needed by the working muscles without raising his heart rate as high as it went when he was untrained. The figure opposite illustrates this principle. All you need to do is perform a standardized bout of exercise for at least three minutes so that the heart rate has a chance to rise up to the level demanded by the exercise, and then measure your heart rate. As you

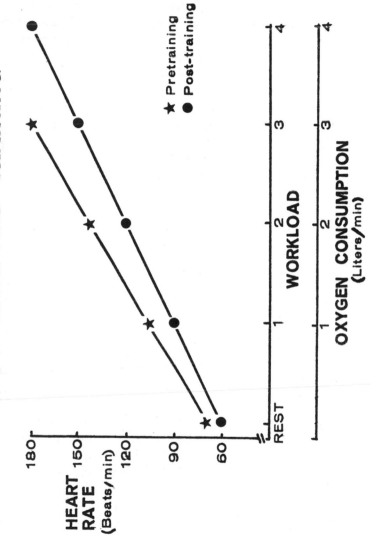

HEART RATE AND TRAINING

★ Pretraining
● Post-training

HEART RATE
(Beats/min)

180
150
120
90
60

REST

WORKLOAD
1 2 3 4

OXYGEN CONSUMPTION
(Liters/min)
1 2 3 4

progress through your fitness program, repeat the test every few weeks to keep track of your progress. You should find that your heart-rate response to the test is reduced progressively as your fitness improves. Incidentally, you'll probably also see your resting heart rate decline as the weeks of training progress, but the resting change is not usually so marked as the one in response to a standard exercise.

One of the easiest types of exercise to use for this test is stepping up and down on the first step of a stairway (these steps are usually eight inches high). A complete step up and down should take two seconds, so you complete 30 steps per minute for three minutes. Upon stopping, locate your pulse immediately, at the wrist or on the neck just alongside the windpipe (press gently on only one side) and at exactly five seconds after stopping count the number of beats for fifteen seconds. This number multiplied by four gives you your heart rate in beats per minute. The reason for taking the heart rate immediately after stopping is that it drops quickly once you stop exercising.

Record in your exercise journal the date and your heart rate in response to the exercise. Remember to keep the stepping rate constant every time you do the test so that the only thing that varies is your heart rate.

In order to be most accurate, the test should bring your heart rate into the range of 120 to 150 beats per minute. While your *resting* heart rate can be influenced by how you feel, how well you slept last night and when you last ate, exercising at a high intensity makes exercise the dominant influence on your heart rate, and other factors become less important. There's no need to bring your heart rate above 150, because then you'd be approaching a maximal effort. If you find that 30 steps per minute on an eight-inch step leads to a heart rate above or below the 120 to 150 range, use a slower or faster rate of stepping.

Your heart-rate response to a standard bout of exercise gives you an indication of your aerobic fitness, but the exact mode of exercise used isn't critical. If you walk, run, cycle or swim for several minutes at a steady pace, using a watch to assure that the exercise intensity is held constant over the course of training, you should see your heart rate decline as the weeks go by. After a while you'll find that this standard work task becomes so easy for you that your heart rate doesn't rise into the 120 to 150 range. Then you need to increase the intensity of the exercise used for the test.

Your heart-rate response may not go down in a systematic way from test to test, due to the various factors that influence heart rate, but in general you should see steady progress, especially in the first several months of training.

Don't confuse the intensity and duration of exercise used in the test with the intensity and duration desirable in the exercise program itself. To give you a record of progress in aerobic fitness, the test exercise must be held constant from test to test, but in your exercise program you should let the exercise become more strenuous—walk or swim faster or longer or both—from week to week to assure that your body is achieving enough of an overload.

Training for Aerobic Fitness

In training for aerobic fitness, you must consider two factors: what type of exercise it should be, and how the overload should be applied —that is, the optimal intensity, duration and frequency.

Although many types of exercise can provide an aerobic training effect, they must engage a large muscle mass continuously for at least five to twenty minutes so that a great deal of oxygen is used, thereby providing a stimulus to the circulatory and respiratory systems. Exercises that meet this requirement include walking, running, swimming, dancing, cycling, basketball, soccer, handball, skiing and racquet sports. Activities such as light calisthenics, yoga, baseball and strength training are usually too localized or sporadic to provide an aerobic training stimulus. The intensity of the exercise should be high enough to stimulate the body but not so high that you grow tired too quickly.

Since the walk-run mode of exercise meets the requirement of engaging a large amount of muscle mass and is a popular aerobic activity, how do you find the most effective intensity of this exercise, with the understanding that the principles may be applied to other activities as well?

There are three techniques you can use to decide how hard you should work. First is the *heart-rate method.* When you walk-run for several minutes at a steady pace, the working muscles need to have oxygen and nutrients brought to them and waste products taken away. In response to this need, the heart beats stronger and faster to pump the needed blood to the muscles. By simply measuring your heart rate you can gain a fairly accurate idea of how intense the walking or running is for you. You should aim to keep your heart rate in the target zone, which is 70 to 85 percent of your maximum heart rate. So if your maximum heart rate is 200 beats per minute (bpm), your target zone is 140 to 170 bpm. A heart rate in this zone indicates that the exercise is stimulating to the physiological systems involved, while being of low enough intensity so that lactic acid does not build up quickly and produce premature fatigue.

In order to apply the heart-rate method, the only figure you need to measure is your *maximum* heart rate. You can measure maximal heart rate by taking your pulse for 15 seconds immediately following an all-out effort of several minutes.

But it is not a good idea to perform such an all-out test at the beginning of an exercise program. You can simply estimate your maximal heart rate rather than measure it directly. This is done by subtracting your age in years from 220, since it has been shown that maximal heart rate tends to decline as you grow older. In the older age brackets, aerobically fit people tend to have higher maximal heart rates than non-fit people. The table opposite provides age-predicted maximal heart rates and target zones for relatively unfit people. As you progress to very high levels of aerobic fitness you can try working closer to the upper limit of your target zone. Keep in mind that your age-predicted maximal heart rate is only an *average* value for someone your age, and that there is considerable variability.

The second technique you can use to decide how hard you should work is the *talk test.* If you can easily maintain a conversation while walking or running, you're probably below the upper limit of the target zone.

In our laboratory, we've found that sedentary people often reach their anaerobic threshold at a walking speed, and that when these people start running, they can hardly lift their legs after sixty seconds. Therefore, it might be necessary to start a "running" program by

Age-Predicted Maximal Heart Rates and Target Zones

Age	Approximate Maximal Heart Rate	Target Zone
20	200	140–170
25	195	137–166
30	190	133–162
35	185	130–157
40	180	126–153
45	175	123–149
50	170	119–145
55	165	116–140
60	160	112–136
65	155	109–132
70	150	105–128

walking and gradually increase your speed until you're running. I always tell people to consider themselves as starting a *locomotion* program: it begins with walking, progresses to faster walking, and may eventually increase to a running speed.

Of course, the talk test only helps you to stay below the upper limit of your target zone; it doesn't tell you whether you're working hard enough to be *in* the target zone. Thus, you can use some combination of the heart-rate method and the talk test: learn to listen to both your circulatory and respiratory systems.

A third way to decide how hard to work might be called the *perceived exertion* method. In our laboratory we routinely ask people to indicate on a scale how hard they *think* the exercise is while we are measuring various physiological functions. We generally find a close relationship between the individual's perception of the exertion and the physiological responses. People who are tuned in to their bodies can probably sense and integrate information from a variety of sources to come up with a rating of physiological strain more accurate than any that can be obtained by even the most sophisticated instruments.

Once the intensity of the exercise is set, you must decide how long to continue at it. Durations as short as five to ten minutes can provide an aerobic training stimulus for people who start off in poor condition. About thirty minutes per session of exercise that causes pounding in the legs seems optimal for many people. Going beyond thirty minutes results in only slightly more of a training effect, as far as aerobic fitness is concerned (though of course it uses more calories), while increasing your chances of suffering an orthopedic problem which might put you out of action altogether. The pounding the legs take in such repetitive activities as running and dancing for more than about thirty consecutive minutes sometimes leads to sore muscles and joints, which are certainly unpleasant and may also be disabling. If you're trying to find a way to build exercise into your life on a long-term basis, you won't want it to result in pain.

If you find it difficult or uncomfortable to work continuously for the entire thirty minutes, you can try alternating work periods and periods of rest or low-intensity exercise. For example, you can usually dance for a few hours without too much fatigue because of the alternating exercise and rest periods involved. Several studies done in my laboratory have found this type of "interval training" to be as effective as continuous training, as long as the total amount of work done in the session is close to that done in continuous training.

The best frequency for aerobic training for adults starting a fitness program seems to be two to four times per week. As with duration, working out more than four times a week may give you a slightly greater training effect, but at the cost of increasing your chances of joint and muscle damage. It appears that your different physiological systems recover at different rates from the overload imposed during the exercise session. Connective tissue in muscles and joints seems to require more recovery time between workouts than does the circulo-respiratory system. During the exercise session energy-yielding processes and breaking down of tissue dominate, while during recovery energy is stored and tissues are repaired.

One way to reduce your chances of incurring joint or muscle soreness is to do somewhat different exercises on consecutive days. If your main activity is running, for instance, but you find that joint or muscle soreness results when you run more than three days per week, try walking, swimming or cycling on the other days of the week. In this way you can overload the circulo-respiratory system every day without overstressing the same joints and muscles. By including several aerobic activities in your weekly schedule, you should be able to work out every day without causing joint and muscle problems.

Flexibility

Unlike other components of fitness, flexibility is not measured by determining how much work you can do. Nevertheless, it's extremely important for optimal physiological and psychological functioning, and may make some indirect contribution to your physical working capacity as well.

Flexibility refers to the range of motion you can go through in the various joints of your body, as well as to the ease and suppleness with which the movements can be made. People commonly lose flexibility as they grow older. This happens as a result of a vicious cycle that often starts in youth, when lack of exercise leads to a restriction in the range of motion through which you use your joints. Joints restricted in their movements for months and years tend to tighten up—that is, the muscles, tendons and ligaments around the joints lose elasticity. Then, any attempt to use those joints causes pain, which in turn discourages further attempts to use the joints. After ten or twenty years of this cycle, the range of movement possible in the affected joints may be minimal. Many of the aches and pains that afflict people as they grow older are attributable to this loss of flexibility.

There are two ways of increasing the range and suppleness of movement. One is by increasing the distensibility or stretchability of tendons, ligaments and muscle connective tissue. (These three types of tissue will be lumped together under the general term "connective tissue.") Connective tissue tends to be distensible but rather inelastic. That is, once it is stretched, it tends not to rebound fully to its prestretched state, so that if you repeatedly stretch it beyond its normal length, the connective tissue will eventually be lengthened on a more permanent basis. The other way to increase your range and ease of motion is to increase your ability to relax the muscles involved. When a movement is limited because certain muscles are in a partial state of contraction, it is possible to improve your flexibility simply by learning to relax those muscles.

To show how these two components of flexibility operate, try the following experiment: stand up and, keeping your legs straight, bend over slowly to touch your toes. When you have gone as far as you can go, relax the muscles at the back of your legs and trunk, and you will find you can bend over a little more.

There are two ways of doing exercises to enhance flexibility: *ballistic* and *static*. A ballistic movement is one in which the body segment is "thrown" so that momentum carries the segment beyond its usual range of motion, as when you touch your toes by thrusting your fingers down forcibly toward them. Although the use of momentum does allow the soft tissues to be stretched more effectively, you can pull or strain a muscle if the movement is too vigorous and you are unaccustomed to it, simply because the speed of the motion might allow the damage to occur before you are able to sense the strain and stop the movement. For this reason, it's better to do flexibility exercises in a static manner: that is, slowly bring the body segment to the limit of its range of motion. At the point where strain is felt, stop and hold it for fifteen to thirty seconds. During this time, make a conscious effort to locate and release any tension limiting the movement. You will usually find it possible to increase the extent of movement slightly. Research has demonstrated that static stretching is just as effective as ballistic stretching in enhancing flexibility, and is less likely to cause muscle soreness. In fact, static stretching is often effective in *relieving* muscle soreness.

When should flexibility exercises be done? The scientific evidence doesn't provide firm guidance on this matter. Some professionals suggest that flexibility exercises precede aerobic exercise. Strictly from the point of view of improving flexibility, it seems most sensible to do the stretching exercises at the end of a vigorous workout. The workout raises body temperature, and warm connective tissue stretches more easily than cold, improving the range of motion in the joints and thus the value of the exercises. In addition, aerobic exercises such as running usually involve repeated contractions within a restricted range of movement, leading to tightness of large muscles. Stretching at the end of the session can help relax the muscles and contribute to overall flexibility.

Assessing Flexibility

Flexibility may be assessed by gently moving to the end of a particular range of motion and recording the position of the body segment involved.

Since back pain is related to lack of flexibility in the muscles behind the thighs (hamstrings) and in the back, you might use the sitting toe-touch exercise, which measures flexibility in this area, as your test. Sit on the floor with your legs extended out straight in front of you. Pull your abdomen in and try to reach your toes with your fingers. Concentrate not on pulling down but on reaching out toward your toes. If you can reach your toes or beyond, your flexibility is satisfactory and you need only be sure that you maintain it. If you cannot, you should try to improve your trunk flexibility, using this test to keep track of your progress.

Keep in mind that there are hereditary differences in flexibility just as in other components of fitness, and you may never be able to touch your toes no matter how much you practice. Use this test as a means of keeping track of your own program of development or maintenance, rather than for comparing yourself with others.

People who start a running program must be especially careful about losing flexibility in the back, hamstrings and calves, since running tends to strengthen these muscles more than it strengthens those in the front of the body. So stretch these areas regularly in order to maintain your flexibility.

Body Composition

It has already been noted that overweight and overfat are not necessarily synonymous. Consequently, to gain some idea of how you stand on this component of fitness, you need an index of your fatness. The eyeball test can give you a gross estimate (stand naked in front of a mirror; if you *look* fat, you probably *are* fat), and changes in how clothes fit, especially around the waist for men and hips for women, can provide information on how you're changing as you alter your lifestyle. Furthermore, if you lose weight, most of it will come from your fat stores, so an accurate scale can be very useful. You must be sure to weigh yourself at the same time of day so that such factors as food and drink consumption and bowel movements are fairly constant. Even then, the errors in most scales, plus day-to-day biological variations, are such that you should average the values obtained over several days rather than expecting to see clear-cut progress on a daily basis. Use the desirable weight tables in the Appendix as a rough guide to what you should weigh.

There are several laboratory and clinical techniques, such as underwater weighing or skinfold measurements, for estimating body fat. A procedure for estimating percent body fat using skinfolds is described in the Appendix on page 181. Simply using a tape measure around several parts of the body (for example, the abdomen, thigh, hips and upper arm) will enable you to monitor your progress in a fat control program. Keep in mind that exercise stimulates growth of trim lean tissue even as it melts away bulky fat, so you will become thinner to a greater degree than is suggested by the scale alone.

How Specific Activities Enhance Physical Fitness

Advocates of particular activities or exercise systems often claim that *their* exercise or sport will improve *all* aspects of health and fitness. Needless to say, you should be suspicious of such claims. However, every form of exercise has *some* value in improving your overall fitness.

Many popular sports (for example, basketball, handball, soccer, racquetball and downhill skiing) stimulate both anaerobic and aerobic energy systems, while also enhancing flexibility. The main problem with competitive sports is that you may push yourself too hard, so stay away from such sports until you build up your fitness base.

Activities that engage a large muscle mass and are carried on for long periods of time (walking, cycling, rock climbing, jogging, swimming and cross-country skiing) are well designed for the development of aerobic fitness. While high-quality singles tennis looks as though it *should* stimulate the aerobic system, studies have failed to show that tennis enhances aerobic fitness, perhaps because for most people the action is not sufficiently sustained.

Swimming is an especially good activity for overweight people, because the water supports the body and the pounding on the legs is eliminated. But because fat people are buoyant, they don't necessarily need to work hard to continue swimming for long periods, so be sure to push yourself sufficiently to obtain a training effect. *Swimming for Total Fitness,* a book by Dr. Jane Katz, provides guidance on how to get the most from this activity.

Cycling, either on the road or on a home stationary model, is also valuable for overweight people because it avoids possibly damaging impact stress on the legs while allowing adequate stimulation of the circulo-respiratory system.

Hiking and cross-country skiing are wonderful ways to spend several hours while using large amounts of calories.

Aerobic dancing is a system which uses the principles of aerobic conditioning in connection with dance steps. It can be effective in providing a training stimulus for the circulo-respiratory system, while also burning up lots of calories. The popularity of this exercise-to-music is truly impressive, and it is undoubtedly making a valuable contribution to the fitness of many people.

Folk, modern, ballet and disco dancing can be effective aerobic stimulants and use up a large number of calories. Of course you must do the dances vigorously in order to gain an aerobic training effect, so take your pulse occasionally during a session to make sure you are in your target zone. Many dance forms can develop several fitness components at the same time, and the enjoyment is heightened by the music and social aspects of dancing.

Calisthenic exercises can develop just about all of the fitness components, if arranged properly. Most calisthenics are basically anaerobic in nature, but by arranging a series of exercises for different parts of the body into a circuit, and moving quickly from one to the other, you can keep the circulo-respiratory system active long enough to improve aerobic fitness. And of course many stretching calisthenics directly improve flexibility and relaxation. But be cautious when using calisthenics, because the body is being placed under unaccustomed stress. Orthopedist Hans Kraus has reported that many people who came to him with orthopedic problems had engaged in the Canadian Air Force exercise program, which uses a high-speed circuit of calisthenics, and had found that the high-intensity exercises were too much for their deconditioned bodies.

What has been said about calisthenics also applies to weight training, with the difference that in calisthenics the weight of the body is used to provide resistance, while in weight training, barbells or plates are lifted. Ordinarily we think of weight training in connection with strength development, but it can also make a modest contribution to aerobic fitness and body composition if the exercises are done with relatively light weights and you move quickly from one exercise to another.

Yoga exercises can be effective for flexibility, relaxation and, to some extent, strength. However, they place little sustained stress on the circulo-respiratory system, and they don't use up large amounts of calories. T'ai Chi Ch'uan is an Oriental system of controlled but continuous exercise designed to use all parts of the body. A thirty-minute routine appears to provide an aerobic training stimulus while also using a substantial number of calories.

To Sum Up

Physical fitness, or dynamic health, is made up of several relatively independent factors, which have to be tested and trained with different types of exercise. You must decide which of these factors are important to you and develop a program focusing specifically on those aspects of fitness. For lifelong health and weight control, high levels of aerobic fitness are important for everyone, and you probably should pay at least some attention to the other elements discussed.

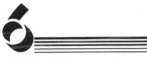

Moving On to Higher Levels: Guidelines and Cautions

By this point you've begun the shift to a high-energy lifestyle. This chapter will outline some general principles of fitness training that you should understand, and will take you through a total exercise session. Later, the hazards that might be associated with your new lifestyle will be discussed.

Training Principles

1. *Your body talks.* Listen to its messages. Ignoring the information your body gives you certainly interferes with the effectiveness of the exercise, and may even cause damage. For example, if you've been running for twenty minutes and your body tells you it's exhausted or in pain, stop or slow down. If you don't, you may injure yourself so that you can't exercise for some time—and you may also come to associate unpleasant feelings of strain and fatigue with exercise.

2. *Easy does it.* The next principle of training is *gradualism.* Improve your physical working capacity a little at a time rather than in large chunks. One of the surest ways to injure yourself is by trying to gain back in two weeks something that you lost over the course of two or twenty years. Many sedentary people who suddenly start exercising

strenuously find themselves flat on their backs. If you establish easily attainable short-range goals and pursue these goals with a modest but effective exercise program, you are likely to succeed—and that success will encourage you to pursue the next short-range goal.

3. *Challenge yourself.* This leads us to the next principle, *progression.* As you achieve each short-range goal, set another that is slightly more challenging. Thus, if you were able to run continuously for fifteen minutes three days this week, you might try to extend the running time to twenty minutes next week.

4. *Know what you're after.* Another training principle is *specificity.* Simply put, this means that you get what you train for. Improving your anaerobic fitness through, say, weight training will not influence your aerobic fitness. The principle of specificity carries over to the part of the body utilized, too, so that exercising your thigh muscles, for instance, won't make your arms stronger.

5. *Push yourself—just a bit.* The *overload* principle of training states that you will develop fitness only if you subject the body to more than the customary effort. If you do twenty-five situps each day, this level of exertion would not constitute an overload, and no further development of abdominal strength and endurance would result if you simply continued to do the same number of situps. However, this degree of exertion would be sufficient to *maintain* your present level of abdominal fitness, which you may find quite satisfactory.

You can increase the overload represented by an exercise by increasing its *frequency, duration* or *intensity.* Frequency can be increased by doing the twenty-five situps twice daily rather than once. You can increase duration by doing thirty situps each time for a while, and then thirty-five, and so on. Intensity can be increased by speeding up the exercise—for example, doing thirty situps in sixty seconds instead of twenty-five situps—or by increasing the resistance overcome by each situp—hold a five-pound weight behind your head while doing them. The unifying concept behind the different ways of altering overload is the *total amount of work done in a given amount of time.*

This concept of work done per unit of time can help us to manipulate the overload of an aerobic activity too, such as running. If you're presently running two miles in twenty minutes on Monday, Wednesday and Friday of each week, you can increase the *frequency* by also running on Tuesdays, Thursdays and Saturdays; the *duration* by running three miles each time; and the *intensity* by doing 2.2 miles in twenty minutes. You can also increase intensity by wearing leg weights while running or by carrying something on your back, but this is not the usual way to increase the intensity of running. The unit of time used may be seconds, minutes, days, hours, or weeks. Indeed, some runners keep track of miles run per month, reaching the desired mileage through various combinations of daily and weekly effort.

6. *Give yourself a rest.* The training principle of *recovery* complements the overload principle. When a particular system of the body is overloaded, the energy-releasing mechanisms are called upon. The body rebounds from such activity with increased energy-storing activity during the recovery period. This energy-storing activity usually continues to a point where the total energy stored is greater than it was before the overload was first applied. For instance, swimming the crawl for thirty minutes will require the use of much of the glycogen in the arm and shoulder muscles. If sufficient recovery time is allowed, perhaps a day or two, and if the proper nutrients are ingested, the amount of glycogen in the arm and shoulder muscles will build up to a level higher than it was before the thirty-minute swim. And if this process is repeated on a regular basis, the muscle glycogen and the work capacity will continue to increase. This is one aspect of the well-known training effect that many people have experienced at one time or another.

7. *Don't lose it!* The last training principle to consider is *regression.* If you allow a long time to pass between workouts, the capacity of the systems *not* being overloaded will diminish. Thus, doing one workout might have a small stimulating effect, but if a week is allowed to elapse before the next workout, the level of fitness will probably regress to what it was *before* the first workout. Another way to look at it is to say that the total work done per month (the overload) resulting from one workout per week is too meager to elicit a training effect.

It's easier to maintain a given fitness level than it is to attain it in the first place. For example, two aerobic workouts per week can maintain a level of aerobic fitness that has taken you six workouts a week for ten weeks to develop. And two anaerobic workouts per week are probably sufficient to maintain anaerobic fitness. Of course, from the point of view of calorie expenditure, you might want to exercise more often.

The Complete Exercise Session

A complete exercise session includes a warmup, a stimulus period and a cooldown. The warmup consists of five to ten minutes of gentle stretching, light calisthenics, and perhaps walking or some other activity that is a modest version of the day's main stimulus activity. The stimulus portion of the workout usually involves fifteen to thirty minutes of more or less continuous aerobic activity. The cooldown usually takes the form of five to ten minutes of calisthenics, stretching and gradual deceleration.

During the warmup phase, the muscles actually warm up: the heat that is liberated increases muscle temperature, which improves the muscle's ability to contract efficiently. The circulatory system is gently stimulated so that the heart rate, cardiac output, circulation to the working muscles, and respiratory apparatus all begin to mobilize to higher levels of function. The cartilage between the bones is thickened by the squeezing and releasing action of exercise, providing more of a cushion between the bones and reducing the friction which might lead to inflammation. People with arthritis or bursitis should be especially careful to warm up gently before exercising.

Perhaps the most important reason for warming up is to overcome inertia. It's hard to get moving from a dead stop, but once you're rolling it's relatively easy to speed up a bit and increase intensity.

Studies of the effect of preliminary exercise on performance show that the warmup is especially useful before activities requiring all-out bursts of speed or power, such as sprinting or jumping events. When the air temperature is very cold or you're going into cold water, it's important to warm up first—particularly for events that require quick contraction of the muscles, such as sprinting or throwing a ball— because the muscles will be rapidly cooled by the air or water, interfering with their efficiency and the speed with which the nerves can transmit the impulses. Nerve conduction velocity is slowed by very low temperatures. If you don't warm up the muscles and the connective tissue, you might tear a muscle.

Aerobic activities of longer duration, however, where the person starts at a submaximal level and gradually builds up speed and intensity, seem to have a warmup built in, and performance isn't improved as much with an extra warmup. In fact, performance in these activities may actually be limited by reaching a certain maximal temperature (the body doesn't function well if the temperature goes up by more than a few degrees), so that it may not be a good idea to increase your body temperature before starting: you're cutting into your maximal capacity.

During the stimulus portion of the workout try to keep the level of work somewhere in the target zone, as measured by the heart rate, the talk test, or the level of perceived exertion. You want to stay within about 70 to 85 percent of maximal heart rate, or above your anaerobic threshold and below the point where talking becomes impossible.

The most important reason for a gradual cooldown is that an abrupt cessation of exercise can cause fainting or dizziness. The total blood volume of the body is insufficient to supply all the muscles and other parts of the body that might utilize blood at the same time. Instead, the body carries a small amount of blood and redirects it where it's needed under various circumstances. When you engage in physical exercise that uses the legs, large amounts of blood are directed toward the leg muscles and away from other organs. This blood brings the necessary oxygen and nutrients, and takes away the waste products and heat. The blood then comes back up to the heart through the veins, from where it is pumped to the lungs for the expiration of carbon dioxide, and the process starts again. The veins are what is called a low-pressure system—that is, the blood pressure in the veins is low compared to that in the arteries. As a result, the blood is helped to return to the heart by the squeezing action of the muscles. When the leg muscles contract, they squeeze the veins which run along them, forcing the blood back up toward the heart. The veins have little valves that prevent the blood from flowing backwards.

If you stopped exercising suddenly, much blood would remain in the legs and not be pumped back up toward the heart. Cardiac output would drop sharply, and the amount of blood going to the brain would be inadequate to maintain consciousness, so you might feel dizzy and faint. If for some reason you do have to stop suddenly, sit or lie down to avoid the possibility of falling down, and try to contract the leg muscles a bit to assist in the flow of blood back to the heart.

Stretching of the muscles that have been used during the stimulus phase is also important during the cooldown, especially if you've been doing an activity that repetitively used the same muscles. Static stretching also assists in relaxing you, and there's no better way to end a session than with a feeling of warmth and relaxation: it's a wonderful way to reinforce the activity. During this period—which can take place lying flat on your back—you might spend a couple of minutes engaging in the relaxation response (see Chapter 7) and thinking about how good your body feels and how great it is to have the power to make yourself feel this way.

The cooldown phase is also a good time to do some of the calisthenics that help prevent back pain and increase muscular strength.

Cautions for the High-Energy Lifestyle

The question of whether you should have a medical examination before undertaking an exercise program is one that has generated a lot of controversy. Some experts recommend that men and women over thirty-five have a medical exam that includes an exercise stress test before starting any exercise program. There is some logic behind this position. A medical exam is a sort of road test: the physician can look at your physiological response to exercise and, if you show no physiological changes that could be interpreted as dangerous, can give you a clean bill of health and permission to exercise at will. But it's not always possible to get completely accurate information from a medical exam. It is possible (though it doesn't happen often) for a person to have a thorough medical exam, complete with stress test, come through it with no indication of problems, walk out the door, start exercising and have a heart attack. On the other hand, it's also quite possible for someone who has clear indications of heart disease to engage in an exercise program with great benefit to his health.

Some physicians and exercise physiologists have taken the position that leading a sedentary life is potentially more harmful to health than leading a high-energy life, and that it's the person who wants to lead a sedentary life who needs a medical exam, to see whether his body can stand the inactivity! If everyone who needed to exercise waited until he could schedule (and afford) a stress test, more harm would probably be done by the resulting inactivity than would occur if everyone went out and exercised as soon as the idea occurred to him or her.

A periodic medical examination and stress test can provide a useful status report for you and your physician on your medical condition. You should at the same time have an ECG and measure your high-density and low-density lipoproteins and triglycerides, and perhaps even your fasting insulin and glucose levels, along with your blood pressure.

Whatever you decide to do about a medical examination, start any exercise program gradually and progress slowly. If you follow this procedure, and at the same time listen carefully to your body, using the guidelines in this book to help you know what to listen for, you will be doing the safest and most effective thing possible for your health. Another excellent reference book to have for your new lifestyle is *The Sportsmedicine Book* by Dr. Gabe Mirkin and Marshall Hoffman. If later on you're interested in the physiological changes that occur (apart from the ones you can readily observe yourself), you can return for a periodic stress test and blood test and a retaking of the tests mentioned above.

Muscle soreness

One of the most common problems of people who are just beginning a high-energy lifestyle is various aches and pains, usually in the legs. This is especially true if you are overweight, because you're carrying that much more of a burden and putting extra strain on the legs. You may also get aches and pains if you haven't been exercising for a while and then resume your routine. Many people think they can simply pick up where they left off, and are very chagrined to find themselves tired and achy for several days.

What should you do if you experience sore muscles the day after strenuous exercise? First, it's important to classify the soreness. If it occurred as a traumatic event (you suddenly felt a tearing or pulling sensation during exercise), it's more likely to be a torn muscle than a sore one, and should be treated with ice to reduce the inflammation and keep down swelling. The same applies to joint sprains or suspected breaks: cease the exercise immediately and apply ice. If ice isn't available, elevate the injured limb to try to reduce the amount of fluid that collects in the area and the resultant swelling. Treat a sprain as if it is a break until the pain subsides. If in doubt, check with your doctor lest you incur permanent damage by using the injured limb.

There are two main theories about muscle soreness that comes on after several hours, or the next morning. One is that the soreness is due to microscopic tears in the muscle or connective tissue; the other is that muscle spasms, interfering with blood flow to that part of the muscle, cause the pain. It's important to distinguish between them, because the treatment for each is different. Try very gently to stretch the sore muscle. If the pain increases markedly, you probably have some torn fibers. If the pain seems to diminish, you may have a spasm.

If you have a muscle tear, treatment with ice for the first twenty-four hours and alternating ice and heat thereafter is called for. Some physicians suggest resting the injured part, and others think that gentle movement will speed the recovery process.

If you conclude that you have a muscle spasm, however, stretching can help to relieve the spasm and hasten recovery. Herbert de Vries of the University of Southern California has performed some experiments which suggest that much muscle soreness is, in fact, due to spasm, and that the use of *static* stretching can be very helpful in reducing spasm and its associated pain.

Exercising in the heat

When we exercise, less than 25 percent of the calories we use up are transformed into the mechanical energy that allows us to use our muscles, and the remaining 75 percent-plus are converted to heat, which must be taken away from the body to avoid dangerous increases in the body temperature. There are four main ways in which this is done: conduction, convection, radiation and evaporation.

Let's see what happens when you're exercising strenuously. If your skin temperature is higher than the air temperature, some heat is conducted from the skin to the environment. Breezes help take the warm air molecules away from the body; convective air currents transfer heat even more quickly. If the sun isn't shining on you (you're not getting radiation from the sun), you will be radiating some heat out into the environment.

If all three of these processes are functioning well, you might find you're not sweating very much; this is often the case when you're working at a moderate level of intensity in a cool environment (which includes in a swimming pool, where conduction and convection work very well in transferring heat to the water). However, if the environmental temperature goes above 90 degrees or so, it begins to approach skin temperature (93 degrees F.), and you progressively lose the ability to transfer heat to the environment through conduction, convection and radiation. If the temperature goes over 93 on a sunny day, you would actually be gaining heat from the environment through these mechanisms, in addition to the heat that your body is generating due to the exercise, and evaporation is the only mechanism left to get rid of heat.

Exercising in a hot, dry environment makes it possible to maintain body temperature because of the ability to lose heat through evaporation. You need to remember, though, that you're losing large amounts of water through evaporation, and that you have to replace it.

When it's hot and humid, however, the ability of the surrounding air to absorb water is diminished, and there's no place for the heat to go. Heat then builds up rapidly in the body, and the body temperature climbs—possibly to an extremely dangerous level. Body temperature has been known to rise as high as 108 or 110 degrees F., which may result in death.

Use your judgment about exercising when the temperature climbs above 90. If you must exercise, wear as little as the law allows, but guard against sunburn. A hat will help protect you. Of course, you can swim without worry no matter how high the temperature, as long as the water temperature is 10 degrees or so below skin temperature and the metabolically produced heat can be transferred to the water.

In both dry and humid conditions, you can lose so much water through sweating that the cardiovascular system doesn't have enough plasma to carry out its various functions, and you experience what is called heat exhaustion: that is, your work capacity becomes limited. Heat exhaustion is characterized by a weak, rapid pulse, cold clammy skin, and sometimes dizziness and fainting. A victim of heat exhaustion should be given rest and as much fluid as he can take. He should be covered with a light blanket, because the skin is cool due to rapid heat loss, and he is in danger of getting chilled. Usually the body temperature has not risen drastically in this type of heat injury.

Heatstroke is a much more serious condition in which the heat regulatory system of the body breaks down. The circulation to the skin is reduced, and much less heat can be taken from the center of the body out to the skin, so the temperature rises very quickly. The symptoms are hot, flushed, dry skin (sweating has ceased), a high temperature (sometimes up to 107 degrees or higher), and delirium. A person with heatstroke needs immediate medical attention. The temperature should be brought down as quickly as possible with cold sponges or a cold bath.

Heat exhaustion and heatstroke can occur when the temperature is not particularly high—even in the seventies—if the relative humidity is extremely high, because so much heat can be generated in strenuous exercise that even in a relatively low temperature a great deal of perspiration needs to be evaporated.

Heat cramps are muscle spasms, usually associated with heavy sweating and fatigue but with a relatively normal body temperature. They're caused by the loss of large amounts of salt through perspiration. If you should engage in strenuous exercise for several days in a row and lose more salt than you are replacing, salting your food more liberally than usual will probably take care of the problem.

The question of exercise and heat has to be considered when you travel from one climate to another. If you live in the North and go to visit a friend in the South, for instance, you might try to continue your usual jogging or walking routine only to find yourself suffering from heat exhaustion. Becoming acclimated to heat takes a few days. The best way is to exercise in the heat—of course at a reduced level. The increase in temperature and heart rate as you exercise will be reduced dramatically over the course of a few days. You'll find your ability to sweat increasing, and as a result you'll get rid of heat much faster, your heart rate won't go so high, and you'll feel more comfortable.

Exercising in the cold

Because your body generates heat to make you comfortable even in cold environments, the chief problem with exercising in the cold is maintaining a balance between the amount of exercise you're doing and the kind of clothing you're wearing. When you first go out into the cold, you usually feel you need heavy clothing, but after you've been moving for a while, you've generated a lot of heat and feel much warmer. Dress, then, in such a way that you feel comfortably warm when you first go out, but can remove some layers after you've started generating heat and tie them around your waist or put them in a backpack. Do some warming up in the house before you go out so that you are able to wear relatively light clothing when you leave the house. Even on cold days, most people find that they work up quite a good sweat and their clothing gets wet. After you finish, go indoors before you become chilled, or put your heavy clothing back on if you remain outdoors.

When it's really cold outside, protect peripheral parts of your body such as your hands and face. Wear knit hats and gloves, and take them off, if necessary, as you get very warm. They can be replaced later.

Don't allow yourself to get caught far from home with inadequate clothing. If you go out for a long vigorous hike, you may feel you don't need warm clothing or raingear, but then find yourself several miles from home, very tired and unable to keep walking rapidly. You may then lose heat to the environment much faster than you can generate it, and it can be dangerous. Experienced hikers always carry raingear to protect themselves from sudden changes in weather. I once learned about this the hard way. My wife and I went on a guided hike wearing shorts and T-shirts—the temperature was in the seventies and we were expecting to walk vigorously. Suddenly it started to pour and the temperature dropped ten degrees. All around us, people were dipping into their backpacks for raingear while my wife and I looked for some kind of shelter. None was available, and were we two miserable people!

Long periods of cold exposure accompanied by low levels of activity —more heat loss than heat production—can lead to hypothermia (*hypo* means under; *thermia* means heat). This reduction in body temperature sometimes occurs after a full day of skiing or hiking. After several hours, there may be glycogen depletion from the muscles, requiring a drop in exercise intensity—that is to say, in metabolic rate. If you're going to be out for a few hours in cold weather, bring along some things to eat: raisins and candy, for instance, can be useful in maintaining the blood glucose level, and thus in maintaining your work capacity. They also serve to increase heat production and keep body temperature stable.

If some part of the body is exposed to the cold, especially in heavy winds, frostbite can occur. Symptoms are numbness in the exposed area and redness progressing to extreme whiteness, meaning that this part of the body is actually frozen and needs immediate attention. Don't rub the affected part or apply snow to it; simply cover it with another part of your body or soak it in warm (not hot) water and allow it to thaw out slowly.

On cold, windy days, set up a buddy system so that you and a companion can observe each other's faces. Sometimes you feel warm enough in general because of your warm clothing and vigorous exercise, so your face doesn't feel uncomfortable even though it may be getting dangerously cold.

Exercising in the water

Water conducts heat away from the body quickly—so quickly that hypothermia can occur any time you're in water below skin temperature. Most people would find extended exposure to water below 70 degrees chilling. Of course, if you're swimming vigorously and generating great amounts of heat, you might find it pleasant to be in water of that temperature. But keep in mind that you're losing large amounts of heat to the water in this kind of exercise, partially because the convective currents caused by your limb movements facilitate heat transfer. Also, the use of your limbs causes blood to be sent to them and more heat can be lost.

Because of the possibility of hypothermia from extended exposure to cold water, avoid swimming by yourself far from a dock or the shore. A process similar to the one discussed in connection with exercising in cold air applies here: the level of heat production you are capable of at the beginning of your swim may be reduced as you become more tired, and you may find yourself unable to maintain body temperature. This can lead to muscle stiffness, making it even more difficult to maintain body temperature, and can cause drowning.

Another problem can occur when swimming underwater. People sometimes try to extend their time underwater by taking a number of deep breaths before diving. There's some danger involved in this, however.

The drive to breathe is mainly determined by a buildup of carbon dioxide in the body fluids. When you take a number of deep breaths (hyperventilate) before diving in, you're washing carbon dioxide from the body fluids—lowering the level. That's why you're able to swim further before you feel the tremendous drive to breathe. But during an extended period underwater the oxygen level in your body can get so low that you pass out and drown. So it's a risky business to hyperventilate too much before swimming underwater, and you should certainly never do it alone.

Exercising at altitude

The main difference between exercising at a high altitude and exercising at sea level is that there is a reduced pressure of all the gases in the air, including oxygen. This means that the air molecules are further apart: if you take a given volume of air into your lungs, you'll be getting fewer molecules of oxygen. Since all gases flow from a higher to a lower level, the reduction in the pressure of oxygen in the air around you means that you'll have reduced oxygen pressure in your lungs, and there will be less of a pressure gradient between the oxygen in your lungs and in your blood. Therefore, the hemoglobin will not become as fully saturated with oxygen as it does at sea level. This in turn will lead to a reduction in the amount of oxygen that can be delivered to the working muscles and other parts of the body, and aerobic working capacity will be reduced.

It's quite common, when you first reach a high altitude, to experience altitude sickness: dizziness, nausea and headache. When you exercise, you'll find you have to take in more air, because each unit of air you take in will have a reduced amount of oxygen. You'll probably also find that your anaerobic threshold will be lower because of the reduction in oxygen pressure. Therefore, you should plan to do less exercise on the first few days at high altitude. After seven or so days at altitude the body adapts in a number of ways to the reduced oxygen pressure, including an increase in hemoglobin concentration. Because each hemoglobin molecule is less likely to be fully saturated, the body adjusts by increasing the number of hemoglobin molecules, thus increasing the total amount of oxygen carried by each unit of blood. However, it doesn't seem possible to reach levels of oxygen consumption and working capacity which are the same as those attained at sea level.

Exercise in polluted environments

More and more people today are engaged in exercise such as walking and long-distance running and bicycling, and in many cities, jogging and bicycling trails run next to highways. Many people wonder whether the pollution created by automobiles makes exercise in these environments unwise. Certainly the carbon monoxide from cars leads to a reduction in the ability of the hemoglobin in the blood to bind with oxygen—that is, carbon monoxide has a greater affinity for hemoglobin than oxygen does. If both are available to the hemoglobin, carbon monoxide will take precedence, crowding out the oxygen. The smog that's found in some of our larger cities also has a variety of pollutants in it, which can damage the pulmonary system.

When you exercise, you're taking in and blowing out much larger volumes of air than you normally do. Therefore, you're taking more pollutants from the air than you normally do. Try to avoid exercising near highways or in polluted areas. Take the extra few minutes to get to a park or an area of town that isn't heavily trafficked. Still, the many benefits of exercise probably outweigh the possible harmful effects of exercising in polluted environments.

7

Staying Healthy

The high-energy lifestyle can do more than just enhance our dynamic health by reducing body fat, improving anaerobic and aerobic fitness, and increasing flexibility. It can actually help prevent illness. This chapter will show you how appropriate exercise and relaxation techniques can reduce stress and tension (and stress-related illness), increase cardiovascular health, prevent back problems, and even slow down the aging processes.

Stress

Stress is the complex of physiological changes that result when you are confronted by a stressor. For example, a large dog suddenly leaping at you constitutes a stressor, and the increase that occurs in your muscle tension and heart rate is part of the stress response.

Stress is by no means a purely negative concept. In fact, we need a certain amount of stress for the body to function properly and to withstand the effects of other kinds of stressors; too little stress can be as damaging as too much. Exercise is a stressor, and many people expose themselves to far less of it than is healthy.

When your body adapts to repeated stimulation with a given stressor, and your response to that stressor is progressively diminished, we have an example of *simple resistance:* you have built up resistance to the stressor. In the case of exercise, this is simply getting in shape, a well-known phenomenon. But the fascinating aspect of stress theory, as first formulated by Dr. Hans Selye, is that at the same time as you are building resistance to exercise, you are building resistance to a wide variety of other stressors as well, a phenomenon that Selye called *cross-resistance.*

To illustrate this concept, Selye conducted a number of rather morbid experiments. In one, rats which had been weakened over a few day's time by treatment with certain chemicals had a leg fractured. The trauma of this injury led to fatal heart attacks in the untrained animals, but not in the rats who had been pretrained with exercise. The exercise training in some way raised the animals' general adaptive abilities, enabling them successfully to withstand sudden exposure to a stressor that killed untrained animals. Dr. N. W. Zimkin and his colleagues in the U.S.S.R. showed that systematic training with exercise also increased the resistance of rats to heat, cold, infections, certain poisons and radiation.

Dr. Ronald Fusco and I investigated the principle of cross-resistance with human subjects. All the college men who served as subjects had their heart rates and blood pressures measured at rest and when one of their hands was immersed in ice-cold water. This localized cold stressor raised their heart rates, systolic blood pressures and diastolic blood pressures (the indexes we used for the stress response) by about 13 beats per minute for heart rate, and 14 and 16 millimeters of mercury for systolic and diastolic blood pressures, respectively. Their heart rate and blood pressure response to a standard bench-stepping exercise was also measured. Next, the subjects were divided randomly into two exercise groups and a control group. One exercise group took part in a ten-week jogging program designed to improve aerobic fitness, and the other did repeated bouts of weight exercises designed to improve anaerobic as well as aerobic fitness. The control subjects took part in a bowling class, an activity not sufficiently intense to stimulate the general adaptive capacities and improve the fitness of most college men. After the training period, the response of the control group to the bench-stepping and cold stressor was unchanged.

But both of the training groups showed a markedly reduced stress response (that is, less of an increase in heart rate and blood pressure) to the bench-stepping, showing improved simple resistance, as well as to the cold stressor, showing improved cross-resistance.

Although the physiological mechanisms behind simple resistance and cross-resistance are incompletely understood, their implications for health are enormous. It is partially through this ability to increase general resistance to stress that exercise improves health and longevity.*

The increase in temperature produced by strenuous exercise may actually boost the capacity of your immune system to resist the ill effects of a wide variety of bacteria. It is already known that fever brought on by a cold or virus can help ward off more serious illness. The virus or bacteria stimulate white blood cells to multiply, and some of these cells go on to produce a small protein called pyrogen. The pyrogen causes the body's temperature to rise, leading to changes in the blood that make it harder for the enemy bacteria to survive.

A 1982 study found that the temperature increase elicited by jogging was also due to pyrogen. People who become regular exercisers often report that they get sick less often than before; perhaps this is due to the pyrogen-temperature mechanism. Dr. Joseph Cannon, one of the authors of the study, took up long-distance running five years ago. "I used to get sick a couple of times a year," he says. "Now it's only once every other year."

So by placing the body under a moderate amount of stress in a regular way, our capacity to withstand a variety of stressors is enhanced. Unfortunately, in our affluent society, the widespread availability of central heating, air conditioning, cars, and elevators has enabled us to avoid exposure to heat, cold and exercise. Ironically, this reduces our general resistance to such low levels that we are in danger

---

*Regular cold baths and sauna baths are also capable of raising the body's general resistance, and many Scandinavians regularly use these techniques together with exercise. However, keep in mind that different stressors can join together in their effect on the general adaptive capacity of the body. So if you have a tough exercise workout and then follow it with alternating saunas and cold showers, as is common in Scandinavia, the total stress on the body may overwhelm its adaptive capabilities, leading to injury, sickness, or even death.

of dying suddenly from unexpected exposure to a intense stressor of some kind. About half of the first heart attacks suffered constitute the first evidence to the individuals that they had any heart disease at all, and many of these attacks are fatal.

Stress, Exercise, and Relaxation

The complex of physiological responses resulting from environmental stressors has also been called the fight-or-flight reaction, since it seems to prepare the body to fight or flee from an adversary or threat. Over the thousands of generations man has been on earth, he has undoubtedly needed this reaction to assure his survival. But now we rarely need to actually fight or flee from an adversary; in fact, in many cases it is out of the question. When your boss causes your heart to pound and your muscles to tense, you ordinarily cannot release the tension by attacking him or running away. Rather, you have to bottle up these impulses. Dr. Herbert Benson, the Harvard cardiologist who wrote *The Relaxation Response,* has suggested that when you are repeatedly exposed to minor stressors, each one of which evokes a minor fight-or-flight reaction, your general physiological state is elevated. For example, after the stress response is provoked, your muscle tension and blood pressure increase. If you actually run or fight, the metabolic products of the exercise cause a relaxation of the muscles and a lowering of the blood pressure. But if you do not fight or flee, the tension and pressure remain high for several hours. If this pattern is repeated every day, your characteristic level of tension and pressure will be elevated. Many of the diseases that have become prevalent in our society in the last generation or so, such as heart disease, high blood pressure, ulcers, colitis, chronic headaches, and chronic back pain, are probably the result of excess tension of this sort.

Exercise, which raises muscle tension and blood pressure to very high levels for a short period, leads to a kind of "rebound" effect in which the tension and pressure levels are actually reduced for the rest of the day. This phenomenon was demonstrated in a study by Dr. Herbert de Vries of the University of Southern California. Dr. de Vries tested a number of elderly men who had high blood pressure and relatively high levels of muscle tension* even when at rest. Tests also showed that these men suffered from a high degree of anxiety, which is often bound up with muscle tension and high blood pressure. Each man had his resting muscle tension determined before and after (1) taking a mild tranquilizer, (2) taking a placebo, (3) walking on a treadmill at a relatively mild pace that elicited a heart rate of about 100 beats per minute, and (4) walking at a pace that elicited a heart rate of 120 beats per minute. The exercise treatments were more effective in reducing tension than the tranquilizer; in fact, the tranquilizer was no more effective than the placebo! Another study showed a marked drop in the resting blood pressure of people with high blood pressure as a result of regularly performing for five to eight weeks a series of isometric exercises, which themselves lead to an increase in pressure during the exercise. And a number of studies have shown that regular endurance exercise leads to reductions in the blood pressure of hypertensive people.

Relaxation Techniques

Exercise can lead to relaxation as a by-product, but you can also relax by more direct action.

A number of techniques have been developed to help people relax, including biofeedback, autogenic training and hypnosis. Edmund Jacobson's progressive relaxation and Herbert Benson's relaxation response can both be learned without the aid of complicated equipment or the presence of a professional. And research has shown both to be very effective in reducing muscle tension and high blood pressure.

Start by practicing the relaxation response, which is designed to promote general relaxation. Then if you find that some residual tension remains, use progressive relaxation to focus on that particular part of the body. Some people find the relaxation response too passive a procedure for them and respond better to progressive relaxation, which is a more active and focused approach.

---

*This was determined with an electromyograph, which measures electrical activity in the muscle. Electrical activity is closely related to muscle tension.

There are four factors involved in eliciting the relaxation response: (1) a quiet environment; (2) a mental device, such as the repetition of a sound, in order to pull your thoughts away from external stimuli or logical thought; (3) maintenance of a passive attitude toward distracting thoughts, and (4) maintenance of a comfortable position to reduce muscular tension.

Sit comfortably in a quiet environment. Lying down is not a good idea because you may fall asleep. Close your eyes. Then focus on some repetitive or constant stimulus, such as some sound, word or phrase. Benson suggests repeating the word *one.* In Transcendental Meditation each person is given his own secret sound to repeat. You may find it effective to concentrate on your breathing, which should be relaxed and regular.

Try to relax all your muscles, from your toes up to your face, and keep them relaxed.

Continue for ten to twenty minutes, opening your eyes to check the time if necessary. Come out of the state gradually when you are finished by sitting quietly for a few minutes with your eyes open and then by stretching your muscles. Do not stand up suddenly, or you may get dizzy due to inadequate blood flow to your head. When you are very relaxed, your blood pressure will probably drop and it needs to rise a bit to support a normal level of activity.

Don't be concerned about being "successful" in eliciting the relaxation response. Try to ignore (without worrying about it) any distracting thoughts by focusing on the word, sound or other mental device you are using. Just keep practicing the procedures one or two times daily and you'll gradually learn to relax more and more completely.

The basic principles of progressive relaxation, as originally set forth by Edmund Jacobson and refined by many others over the last fifty years, are also simple.

Adopt a comfortable position in an armchair or recliner, so that most parts of your body are supported. Alternately tense and relax all parts of the body, generally progressing from the toes to the legs to the trunk, and ending with the neck and the facial muscles. Each time, gradually bring the tension up to high levels, hold it for several seconds or until you experience some discomfort in the contracting muscles, and release it gradually.

There are two rationales underlying this procedure. First, you will find that as you tighten your muscles you will gain greater awareness of muscle tension, thereby allowing you to focus on it and control it. Thus you will be able to modulate it from very high to very low levels. Second, the body has built-in dampening mechanisms for any of its activities. Thus as you forcibly contract a muscle an inhibitory nervous stimulus is sent to that muscle which tends to make the muscle relax. Of course, if you voluntarily continue to contract the muscle, you can usually override this inhibitory stimulus. But if you voluntarily *cease* further contractions, the inhibitory stimulus will bring the muscle to a deeper level of relaxation than would have been possible without the preceding contraction.

After each contraction relax the whole body for ten to twenty seconds and try to sense the tension draining out.

A complete relaxation procedure, which proceeds slowly from toes to head, with ten to twenty seconds between contractions, and finishes with five to ten minutes of total body relaxation, should take approximately twenty to thirty minutes. If you do this once a day you will find yourself becoming more and more effective in achieving a very relaxed state. Even when it is not possible to engage in total body relaxation procedures, your increased awareness of the tension-relaxation continuum will allow you to perform *differential* relaxation, in which you carry out a task using only the necessary muscles while relaxing the rest of the body.

A good time to engage in relaxation exercises is at the end of the workday. Relaxing after an exercise workout is especially easy, since the exercise itself tends to promote relaxation. The pleasant feelings you will experience will also tend to serve as a reinforcement for the whole workout, making it more likely that you will engage in the whole process regularly. But there is no one time that is best for all people. Whenever you feel tension building up you might try to take a relaxation break.

In fact, you might relax in anticipation of tension. By assuring that your muscles are relaxed you can reduce the anxiety you usually experience in certain situations or with certain people. Muscle tension seems to be so central to anxiety that a powerful principle has evolved: *It is impossible to be anxious and relaxed at the same time.*

Cardiovascular Health and Disease

Most adults are aware of the importance of the heart in maintaining life. Unfortunately, many people learn the precise functions of the cardiovascular system from a hospital bed or in a doctor's consultation room. Wouldn't it be better to learn about cardiovascular function *before* trauma occurs, so you can take positive steps to develop a healthy heart? This section will describe cardiovascular function and the effects of exercise or inactivity on the heart and circulatory system. You will find out that you can markedly reduce your chances of being struck down by cardiovascular disease if you adopt appropriate exercise and relaxation behaviors.

Diseases of the heart and circulation are the cause of more than 50 percent of all deaths in the United States. About a million people suffer heart attacks each year, perhaps half of them fatal. For many of these men and women, the first symptom of heart disease is the attack itself. Clearly we have an epidemic in our nation, the result not of some virulent infection spreading through the population, but of our lifestyle.

The two main categories of cardiovascular disease are *coronary heart disease (CHD)* and *hypertension* or high blood pressure. The heart is basically a pump that circulates blood, supplying all parts of the body with life-sustaining oxygen and other essential nutrients. If the pump is weak, oxygen will be denied to organs and muscles, and problems will result. Since the heart muscle itself depends on oxygen, it cannot function properly if the coronary circulation, which feeds oxygen to it, is impaired. The accumulation of fatty substances such as cholesterol in the walls of the coronary arteries over many years progressively narrows the diameter of the blood vessels and reduces the coronary blood flow to the heart muscle. This accumulation of fat hardens into *atherosclerotic plaques,* and the entire process is called atherosclerosis. Suppose a person who has clogged arteries but doesn't know it does something that requires hard physical labor. His muscles are working harder and need more oxygen, so the heart beats faster and harder to circulate more blood. As a result, the heart muscle itself needs more oxygen, but the clogged coronary arteries can't supply fresh oxygen-carrying blood fast enough.

A circulating clot or a small segment of an atherosclerotic plaque that breaks off can get caught in a narrowed section of artery. This coronary thrombosis cuts off the blood supply to the heart muscle fed by that vessel. The imbalance between oxygen demand by the heart muscle and oxygen supplied by the coronary vessels may lead to a *myocardial infarction,* the technical name for the death of muscle tissue due to inadequate oxygen.

There are many cases of sudden death in which some malfunction of the heart is suspected, but in which no infarction seems to have occurred. It is theorized that the inadequate supply of oxygen leads to cardiac arrhythmias in which the different parts of the heart muscle do not contract in proper sequence. These arrhythmias in turn lead to *ventricular fibrillation,* a condition in which the ventricles beat very rapidly (perhaps three hundred times per minute instead of the normal sixty to ninety) and in such an uncoordinated way that almost no blood can be pumped out. Within minutes the stricken person loses consciousness and dies due to inadequate blood supply to the brain and the heart muscle itself. The term *heart attack* is a general layman's term for any sudden, incapacitating event, such as a myocardial infarction or ventricular fibrillation. *Angina pectoris* is the technical term for pain or pressure in the chest or left arm brought on by exercise, cold exposure, or excitement; it is probably the result of inadequate oxygen supply to the heart muscle.

Hypertension is incompletely understood. Although the causes for most hypertension are obscure, it is clear that the higher one's blood pressure, the greater the risk of CHD and the greater the possibility of incurring a stroke due to a broken blood vessel supplying the brain. Millions of people have high blood pressure but are not aware of it because it has no clear-cut symptoms. It is often discovered during routine checkups of apparently healthy adults.

Although the exact causes of CHD are not clear, there are a number of risk factors associated with the disease; that is, people with one or more of these factors are more likely to be struck by CHD during a given number of years than people without the same factors. These risk factors include aging, being male, having high blood pressure, having a high cholesterol level, smoking cigarettes, having a family history of CHD, having diabetes, exhibiting type A behavior,* and living a sedentary life style.

Obesity by itself is not a risk factor, but it contributes strongly to high blood pressure, cholesterol and diabetes. In fact, avoiding overweight is one of the best ways to reduce your risk of CHD. Recently it has been shown that people who put on their excess weight as adults have a much greater incidence of cardiovascular and metabolic disease than those who were also fat as children. Adult-onset obesity is often found in muscular people who become inactive as adults after active childhoods. Their excess fat tends to collect on the trunk of the body, while for childhood-onset obesity more fat collects on the limbs.

Even more striking than the connection of the other risk factors to CHD is the way in which they *multiply* the risk of CHD when they appear together. The result is that individuals with all of the factors present may have a risk of CHD twenty to thirty times as great as people without any of the factors.

Exercise and CHD

The ways in which regular exercise improves cardiovascular health and reduces the risk of CHD may be broadly classified into three areas: (1) modification of risk factors; (2) direct effects on the heart and its circulation; and (3) effects on other organs and systems which in turn influence CHD risk.

Modification of Risk Factors Through Exercise

1. *High blood pressure.* Although the exact cause of high blood pressure is not fully known, we do know some of the factors associated with it. Repeated elicitation of the stress response throughout the day, without an opportunity to release the resulting tensions, can lead to increased blood pressure. Regular exercise discharges tensions, with a subsequent reduction of blood pressure in people with high levels. The relaxation response or progressive relaxation also seems to lower

---

*Behavior characterized by extreme competitiveness and excessive time urgency.

both muscle tension and blood pressure. The type A behavior pattern is characterized physiologically by both high muscle tension and high blood pressure. Thus regular exercise and the use of relaxation techniques may reduce the risk associated with hypertension and type A behavior.

2. *Cholesterol.* Cholesterol, an oily substance called a lipid, is carried in combination with blood proteins, forming lipoproteins. These lipoprotein molecules vary in density, with those having greater amounts of lipid being less dense (just as oil is less dense than water). Most of the cholesterol is carried with low-density lipoproteins (LDL), but about 20 percent is carried in the form of high-density lipoproteins (HDL). While high concentrations of LDL are positively associated with coronary heart disease, those people with high concentrations of HDL tend to have less coronary heart disease. Young women, who have a low incidence of heart disease, have much higher levels of HDL and a much lower concentration of LDL than middle-aged men, who have a high incidence of heart disease.

One of our current studies is comparing active and inactive middle-aged men on a variety of CHD risk factors. The active men have a total cholesterol count of 177 mg per deciliter of blood, compared to 242 mg for the sedentary men. In addition, about 36 percent of the cholesterol is carried in HDL for the active men, whereas in the sedentary men, only 21 percent is carried in this form. The ratio between total cholesterol and HDL cholesterol seems to be the best index of coronary heart disease risk. In our study, this ratio is 70 percent higher in the inactive men. The sedentary subjects have 30 percent body fat, compared to 10 percent for the active men, and this difference in fat is the best predictor of the total cholesterol/HDL ratio. This illustrates the intimate connections between body fat, CHD, and a low-energy lifestyle.

Other studies have shown that middle-aged male runners have ratios that closely resemble those of young women, and that regular exercise or weight reduction tends to shift the ratios in the right direction in overweight males who have low HDL and high LDL concentrations. The effects of weight loss and aerobic training are not so clear in females, perhaps because females tend to have more favorable ratios to begin with. In fact this difference between males and females may help account for the fact that females have a much lower incidence of heart disease.

It appears that HDL carries cholesterol away from the coronary arterial linings to organs like the liver, where it can be metabolized, acting as a kind of scavenger, whereas LDL more rapidly gives up its cholesterol to the arterial walls, hastening the development of atherosclerosis. Total cholesterol in the blood is a less important factor than the proportions of LDL and HDL.

Regular endurance exercise appears to alter the lipoprotein pattern so as to reduce the risk of CHD. It doesn't take massive amounts of exercise. One of my students recently showed that four months of even the modest amount of aerobic exercise that cardiac patients are able to do resulted in significant changes in this ratio. A vigorous walking program has also led to marked changes in the ratio after four months.

3. *Smoking.* Cigarette smoking does not appear to be directly influenced by exercise per se. But few people who exercise regularly continue to smoke, and many stop smoking when they adopt regular exercise habits. One large group of middle-aged runners studied contained no smokers, but half of them were former smokers. Possibly the relaxation elicited indirectly by exercise, or directly by practicing the relaxation response, reduces the need for the relaxation that many smokers derive from cigarettes.

Effects of Exercise on the Heart and Its Circulation

Regular endurance exercise does enhance cardiovascular health. One series of changes that takes place in the skeletal muscles doesn't *appear* to be connected with cardiovascular health, but a closer look reveals some interesting connections. Endurance training increases the oxidative capacity of the trained muscles: that is, the ability of the muscles to liberate energy through aerobic processes is enhanced. When the aerobic capacity of the muscle is insufficient and some of the energy must be liberated through anaerobic pathways, the end product is lactic acid, which accumulates in the muscle and eventually interferes with muscular contraction and relaxation. An increase in the oxidative capacity of the muscle, then, leads to less formation of lactic acid and enhanced work capacity. But what has this to do with the cardiovascular system? The lactic acid sets in motion a set of chemical processes that culminate in a higher heart rate, requiring the heart to work harder. This is one of the ways in which aerobic training leads to a lower heart rate during a standard amount of exercise.

Many of the changes related to cardiovascular health take place in the heart and blood vessels themselves. The clearest effect of endurance training is a reduced heart rate at rest and during a standard work task. Even though the heart rate rises during the exercise session, it is much lower the rest of the day. Fit people may have resting heart rates as low as 40–50 bpm.

The most important factor contributing to the lowered heart rate is the improved pumping action of the heart muscle. Regular endurance exercise increases the pumping power of the heart muscle, with the result that more blood is pumped out with each beat and fewer beats are necessary to pump out a given amount of blood. Along with the improved pumping action goes an increase in the coronary circulation capacity of the heart muscle, permitting delivery of the oxygen so vital to its function, especially at high work intensities or during periods of stress.

A number of animal studies have shown that when atherosclerosis is simulated by artificially narrowing the coronary arteries, and the animals are then subjected to regular aerobic exercise, the collateral blood flow is increased by 400 to 600 percent. Such improved circulation due to exercise has not yet been conclusively demonstrated in human hearts, but this may be due to the relatively insensitive and indirect techniques which must be used in human studies. Since most Americans probably have some degree of atherosclerosis building up as they age, these animal studies may well illustrate the role that exercise actually plays in the adult human.

Another change elicited by training is a reduced tendency of the blood to clot during periods of stress. To some extent, atherosclerosis is a result of small clots being deposited on the inner walls of the coronary arteries, so the reduced clotting tendency may be another factor protecting the active person from heart disease.

The result of the changes caused by endurance training is a reduced tendency to suffer from a lack of oxygen and all of the consequences that follow. Even if some of the heart muscle should be deprived of adequate oxygen, the trained heart will have sufficient pumping power left in the unaffected muscle to allow circulation of sufficient blood to sustain life. In the same situation, the untrained heart might fail and the person die. There is evidence that even when the untrained person survives, it takes him a longer time to recover his ability to function normally.

Active People Get Less Coronary Heart Disease

Many studies have shown markedly less CHD among active than among inactive people. In a study done by Dr. Ralph Paffenbarger and colleagues, 3,606 longshoremen were divided into high- and low-activity groups based on the energy they used during a normal working day. Some of the men did light machine work and others did heavy work like lifting, toting and stacking. Dr. Paffenbarger followed these men over a twenty-year period and kept track of the numbers of fatal heart attacks in both groups. Overall, the low-activity group had 60 to 80 percent more fatal heart attacks than the high-activity group. The difference was most striking when the men were between the ages of thirty-five and fifty-four: the incidence of fatal heart attack was three times as great in the low-activity men. Even when other risk factors, such as heavy cigarette smoking or above-average blood pressure, were taken into account, the role of physical exertion remained dominant. Paffenbarger estimated that if the three main high-risk characteristics had been eliminated, the rate of fatal heart attack would have been reduced by 70 to 100 percent!

In another study, Paffenbarger and associates studied alumni of Harvard University and the University of Pennsylvania. The men who exercised regularly in their leisure time had a rate of heart disease about 80 percent lower than their less active former classmates, and again, the differences were especially striking in the younger groups.

Recently it was shown that jogging prevents coronary heart disease in monkeys. Dr. Dieter Kramsch and colleagues at the Boston University Medical Center taught monkeys to run on a special treadmill for an hour three times a week, and followed their progress for three years. During the last half of this period they were fed an atherogenic diet (one high in butter and cholesterol). The trained monkeys were compared to a group of sedentary monkeys fed the atherogenic diet, and to a third group of sedentary monkeys fed the usual diet of monkey chow.

The trained monkeys developed high levels of total blood cholesterol on the atherogenic diet, as did the sedentary monkeys on the same diet, but the trained monkeys had higher HDL levels and lower triglycerides. Signs of manifest heart disease, including electrocardiographic abnormalities and narrowed coronary arteries, were found only in the sedentary group on the atherogenic diet. The trained monkeys had much less development of atherosclerosis, and their coronary vessels were much wider.

Thus even though exercise did not keep the atherogenic diet from raising total cholesterol levels, the higher HDL and lower triglycerides apparently retarded the development of CHD.

Dr. Kramsch recently came to Columbia University to talk about his research. Some of the monkeys that had developed atherosclerosis from the combination of sedentary living and the atherogenic diet were started on a gradual jogging program for twenty-four months, to see whether the atherosclerotic process could actually be reversed, even though the monkeys continued to eat the high-fat diet. Not all the monkeys became good runners, but atherosclerosis diminished markedly as aerobic fitness improved (as measured by resting and exercise heart rates).

Dr. Kramsch emphasized that this study is not conclusive because of the small number of monkeys involved. But he also emphasized that of all the studies done to date, including those which have tried various diets and drugs, this one showed the most clear-cut reduction of fat and connective tissue in the arteries. Remarkably, it was accomplished by low-intensity exercise for only an hour a day, three times a week, while the monkeys continued to eat a high-fat diet.

While generalizing from one species to another is always risky, there is cause to hope that *atherosclerosis may be not only prevented, but to some extent reversed, through the adoption of a high-energy lifestyle.* Clearly we do not need to accept heart disease as an inevitable consequence of reaching our forties and fifties if we adopt appropriate health habits. And regular aerobic exercise is the most important of these health habits. This was the main conclusion of a multifactorial computer analysis of hundreds of scientific studies on causes of heart disease by Forrest Blanding, as described in his 1982 book, *The Pulse Point Plan*. He found that the incidence of coronary heart disease among people of high aerobic fitness is only 20 percent that of inactive persons, and that the incidence of sudden coronary death is 5 percent that of inactive persons.

Diabetes can also be influenced by lifestyle, a subject that will be discussed in Chapter 10.

Exercise and Back Trouble

Almost everyone has a back problem at some time in his or her life. Although back problems are seldom fatal, they are certainly one of the major health problems in our society in terms of discomfort, time lost from work, and financial cost.

A study by Dr. L. Hult showed that by the age of sixty, 75 percent of a group of 1,200 males showed some subjective symptoms of back trouble and 90 percent showed some objective signs of spinal disc degeneration on an X-ray. Overweight people are especially susceptible to back trouble because of the extra pressure imposed by the excess weight. Again, back trouble is related to our health habits rather than to some organic or infectious disease we cannot control.

Dr. Hans Kraus, an orthopedist, has organized back-pain clinics at New York and Columbia Universities. He found that over 80 percent of the people who came to the clinics had no organic or structural basis for their pain. (Keep in mind that only relatively serious cases were referred to the clinics, and that if all people who at one time or another suffer from back pain were considered, the percentage with an organic or structural basis for their pain would probably be less than 10 percent.) Instead, the pain was due to muscular weakness and/or inflexibility.

The typical person with back pain has tight muscles in the back of the legs and trunk, and weak abdominal muscles. Although the exact causal sequence for back pain is not well understood, Dr. Kraus believes that our tendency to be overstressed and underexercised is to blame.

The stress response includes a tightening of the back and neck muscles. If this occurs many times during a typical day, without the opportunity to release the tension, a high degree of residual tension builds up. When a muscle contracts, it raises its internal pressure to a point where it may exceed the pressure of blood flowing into it. As a result, blood flow is hindered or cut off, leading to a lack of oxygen, pain, and, if carried on long enough, death of some muscle tissue. Sometimes the pain is not confined to the back if some of the nerves leaving the spinal cord are affected, and the person experiences radiated pain in the legs or arms. Even if no serious pain occurs early in life, the stage may be set for problems later on.

As a person ages, the back muscles tighten even more, while inactivity leads to a progressive weakening of the abdominal muscles. The combination of these two factors leads to a downward rotation of the front of the pelvis, best exemplified by the potbellied and swaybacked posture prevalent in middle-aged people. To keep from falling forward on his face, the person must shift the top part of the body to the rear, thereby accentuating the curvature in the lower back. This puts added stress on the rear parts of the spinal discs and causes them to wear out prematurely. If any of the nerves leaving the spinal cord (for example, the sciatic nerves, which run down the outside of the legs) are pinched as a result, the pain can be quite severe. The swaybacked posture is accentuated in people with a lot of excess fat stored in the abdominal area: in order to maintain balance, they have to increase the curvature.

Weak abdominal muscles can have another important consequence, since these muscles indirectly assist the back muscles in many lifting activities. When a person bends forward and lifts a moderately heavy object with his arms, the mechanical levers are such that tremendous stress is placed on the lower back, far more than the back muscles could handle alone. But if the person contracts his abdominal muscles strongly, he makes his trunk into a rigid cylinder and takes much of the strain off the back muscles. If his abdominals are weak, he may seriously strain his back. This is why you should try to lift objects by keeping them as close to the body as possible and by using your leg muscles to a greater extent.*

The lesson is clear: maintain strong abdominal muscles and flexible back muscles throughout your life, and don't get fat.

Exercise and Cancer

Not much research has been done on the relationship between physical activity and cancer, but some evidence suggests that regular exercise might reduce your chances of contracting the disease. As long ago as 1921, a study of over 86,000 men showed that the death rate from cancer was lower in those with jobs requiring more muscular effort. A number of experiments have shown that tumor growth is inhibited in exercising animals who have been subjected to carcinogenic agents. And a study published in 1981 by Dr. Victoria Persky and colleagues showed that higher heart rate was a risk factor for lung and colon cancer in men studied for five to eighteen years. We have seen that aerobic training leads to low heart rates.

The physiological mechanisms underlying these relationships are still unknown. Perhaps the general increase in resistance to stressful agents, discussed earlier, helps the body fight cancer-provoking agents.

Aging and Exercise

Aging is accompanied by the diminution of many physiological capacities. A recent study by Dr. G. W. Heath and colleagues at the Washington University School of Medicine concluded that aerobic fitness declined about 9 percent per decade after age twenty-five in healthy American men. However, about half of this was due to the decreased physical activity and increased body fat which accompanied growing older. Men who maintained their activity and leanness lost only about 5 percent per decade. The major factor responsible for the decline in active men was the reduction in maximum heart rate.

---

*Many back injuries seem to occur when a twisting action is combined with the lift, so avoid turning and lifting at the same time.

Anaerobic fitness (strength and local muscular endurance) declines gradually with age, but the rate of decline is much greater from sixty to ninety than from thirty to sixty. Some of this decline is due to decreased levels of testosterone. This hormone plays a role in protein synthesis, and if it is not secreted in adequate amounts, the muscles get smaller and weaker. But when a group of machine workers who were involved in daily arm exercise were studied, no decline in strength was found between twenty-two and sixty-two years of age, so the age-related decline in fitness may be due largely to disuse rather than to aging per se.

Coordination of complex movements becomes somewhat poorer as we age, leading to a loss of efficiency in movement. There's a reduction in the speed with which the central nervous system is able to process information: the quality of thought and action may be retained, but it will be slower, especially when very complex movements have to be made. Performance in events requiring quickness and power usually suffers. The individual may also find it more difficult to protect himself against injury in fast-moving sports, because he can't make the lightning-quick adjustments required. However, improvement in strategy and anticipation of the other players' movements can allow older people to compete quite successfully with younger ones in many sports.

Flexibility tends to decrease with age, especially in movements which are not practiced. Changes in the connective tissues make them less pliable. In addition, the disease of arthritis becomes more prevalent with aging. This inflammation in the joint causes resistance and pain when the joint is moved. In the acute phase of the disease, rest is necessary to let the inflammation subside. After the acute phase has passed, gentle movement is needed to increase the range of motion and prevent further deterioration of the muscles.

Exercise can reverse the loss of flexibility associated with aging. Dr. Kathleen Munns tested twenty people aged sixty-five to eighty-eight on flexibility in six parts of the body. After twelve weeks of a carefully designed exercise and dance program, all six measurements showed improved flexibility, and the people said that their daily-life movements were more comfortable.

Osteoporosis is decreased mineral mass and strength of bone (15 to

30 percent is lost by age seventy), which leads to a fifty-fold increase in the incidence of hip fracture between ages forty and seventy. Bone is like other tissue: it adapts to stress by increasing mass and strength; when unstressed, it atrophies.

Astronauts suffer mineral loss (mainly calcium) from the bones in just a few days of weightlessness, and the same thing occurs in bed rest. Active workers and athletes have thicker bones than others, indicating the importance of exercise in retaining bone density. Dr. Everett L. Smith of the University of Wisconsin showed that people sixty-nine to ninety-five years of age who exercised three times weekly increased their bone mineral content, while a control group suffered a significant loss of minerals in the three-year period. The mechanisms are not entirely clear. Exercise may result in increased circulation to the bones; increased gravitational and muscular stress may cause electrical activity in the bone which in turn stimulates mineral deposition.

Clearly the rate of the physiological decline that occurs with aging, as well as the level of function, can be altered markedly by use or disuse. And there is certainly much evidence accumulating that most people who exercise regularly lead longer, healthier and fuller lives. The studies of Dr. Herbert de Vries and colleagues have shown that people in their seventies who begin exercise programs can improve their dynamic health to the point where it resembles that of younger people. Cardiologist Lenore Zohman, Jeffrey Young, and I recently collaborated in a study of an eighty-year-old marathon runner, Noel Johnson. We tested him for cardiovascular function and body composition and found his treadmill performance to be as good as that of the average man half his age.

In light of the ability of older people to maintain fairly good aerobic and marathon performance, it seems logical for people to shift gradually towards this kind of activity as they age, participating less in basketball, soccer, handball and other fast-moving, strenuous activities that require great power and involve contact with others, and more in activities like walking, jogging, cycling, swimming, and cross-country skiing.

The bottom line on aging is whether high-energy living actually lengthens life. While controlled experiments cannot be done with humans, a study by Dr. Ernest Retzlaff and colleagues showed that daily exercise increased the lifespan of albino rats by 34 percent as compared to their nonexercised littermates.

So much for our physical well-being. Now let's look at how high-energy living affects our state of mind.

8

A Sound Mind

When you take charge of your exercise habits, your nutritional habits, and your ability to relax, you have your health and happiness to a large extent under your own control. Your body and your mind will be sound and healthy. One of the foremost exponents of this holistic point of view is George Sheehan, the cardiologist who has become one of the major voices in the exercise movement. He has argued that you can't change your body without changing your total being. And it's difficult to change your psychological functioning without having it affect your body in some way. When you feel better physically, you feel better psychologically. And when you feel better psychologically, your body functions more efficiently.

Exercise and Happiness

What is psychological well-being or happiness, and how can exercise or weight control affect it? What makes people happy, anyway? We integrate many kinds of information about our lives in deciding whether we're happy or not. Our answers can refer to how we feel at the moment or to how things have been with us in general over the last few days, weeks or months. Let's look at some of the factors that can keep us from being happy, and then see how exercise affects these obstacles to our psychological well-being.

External realities can interfere with our happiness. "I lost my job and I'm very unhappy and worried." "My wife left me and things are very bad with me these days." "I had a fight with my neighbor." "I'm having problems with my kids." If we can see a solution to the problem, we are less unhappy than if we feel helpless to change the situation.

Our various physiological sensations, too, can prevent us from being as happy as we should be. A person suffering back pain, for example, who finds it very difficult to move at all, let alone do any kind of exercise or work without agony, will certainly be at least somewhat unhappy. We often feel tired, lethargic, out of shape, physically tense. We have headaches and digestive upsets. Maybe we're suffering from some degenerative disease. And the various aches and pains which we often experience as we grow older can affect our state of mind negatively, though many of these are really due to a lack of flexibility rather than to any pathologic problem, and can be helped by exercise and relaxation. Again, if we feel there's a cure for what ails us, we're considerably less unhappy than if we feel we have no control over our pain or illness.

Finally, psychological factors can make us deeply unhappy. Maybe we feel anxious all the time, or have periods of acute anxiety and don't understand why. Maybe we find ourselves being hostile to people without any apparent reason and then feeling guilty. Maybe we're depressed, feeling helpless to alter things around us or our own perceptions of them. When we feel confident of getting better, we automatically feel somewhat better already.

As we look at the range of external realities, physical sensations and subjective feelings that can keep us from being happy, it becomes clear that the less we feel in control of our lives, the unhappier we are. No matter what is bothering us, if we feel that it is in our power to do something about it, our state of mind immediately improves. It's when we feel that we have no control over ourselves and our lives that we become deeply depressed.

The role that exercise can play in all this is to enhance our feeling of potency to control our own lives. Unfortunately, we can't control *all* the factors that influence our health and happiness, but what we *can* change profoundly is what probably has the most important effect on our mental and physical well-being: our own behavior.

Here's what happens: as you engage in exercise, you control your weight more effectively, you improve your appearance, you improve your physical fitness. All these changes lead to increased self-esteem and a feeling of potency and control over your life. These in turn lead to a decreased sense of helplessness and a decrease in depression and anxiety.

As far as external factors are concerned, exercise may not keep you from losing your job, but it can make you a more energetic and efficient worker and therefore more valuable to your employer—and if you do get fired, it can help you avoid depression and give you the vigor to actively seek another job. Maybe exercise won't prevent your spouse from leaving you, but because it makes you feel better about yourself, it can make you a more pleasant person to live with (particularly if the two of you start exercising together)—and if your marriage does break up, you'll be fit, attractive and self-confident when you start dating again.

Exercise is extremely effective in preventing or ameliorating many of the physical conditions that negatively affect our state of mind. Because it makes your heart and circulation work more efficiently, it can help prevent heart attacks and strokes and help cardiac patients recover more quickly. Because it strengthens your muscles, it can prevent back trouble. Because it keeps you flexible, it can help prevent the stiffness and joint problems that otherwise come with age. Because it relieves tension, it can prevent or ameliorate tension-related headaches and digestive problems. There's even some preliminary evidence that it may help prevent cancer.

Exercise as Therapy

Many psychiatrists and psychologists have recognized that exercise has an effect on psychological health as well. In fact, a number of them have taken to using exercise as a form of psychotherapy, especially for depression. One study done by Dr. John Greist and colleagues at the University of Wisconsin compared running as therapy for depression with two other types of depression therapy ordinarily given in their clinic. The subjects ran or walked three times a week for thirty to forty-five minutes each time. The researchers found that of the eight patients who were engaged in this exercise therapy, six were essentially well within three weeks and remained well for the duration of the active treatment. A seventh patient, who didn't start her walking program until the sixth week of the study, recovered after about sixteen weeks. The eighth patient took part conscientiously in all of exercise but showed neither improvement nor deterioration in her depressed condition during the ten-week period of treatment, although she did increase her level of physical fitness. The therapists followed these people up after one year, and found that the results were retained at least for that period of time. They concluded that these results were comparable to the results obtained in ordinary kinds of psychotherapy.

Thaddeus Kostrubala is a San Diego psychiatrist who has written extensively about the value of exercise to psychological health. In his book, *The Joy of Running,* he tells of his personal awakening at the age of forty-two. Even though he was a successful psychiatrist, he had not taken charge of his personal well-being. He was out of shape, unhappy and fearful. In his words, "I didn't have to think very deeply or develop any insight to realize that I was a prime candidate for a heart attack. I weighed 230 pounds. I drank heavily. I did not exercise; I didn't even take walks. I *never* ran. My blood cholestrol was quite high, and my blood pressure was beginning to rise. According to everything I knew about heart disease, I was in line to have a coronary."

Kostrubala started exercising in a program for cardiac patients. The first day he couldn't run a hundred yards. After a few months, he was able to run three miles without stopping. "Three miles! My God, that was an unbelievable distance. I was glowing like a kid who's won some super-special trophy. I told everybody. I guess I was telling everyone else because I couldn't believe it myself. Somehow, if I told them, it would really be real. Running that three miles in the rain remains with me as one of the major beautiful memories in my life." Clearly, his enhanced physical capacity was critical to his mental health.

Not only has Kostrubala become a marathon runner and taken control of his health and well-being, but he uses running in his therapeutic practice. He tells of many cases in which his patients have used running as part of their therapy. The patients' increased feeling of potency helps them to deal more confidently and competently with their social and psychological problems.

Although Kostrubala focuses on running, many other types of exercise can undoubtedly have the same value.

Another psychologist who regularly uses exercise as therapy is Dr. Alan Gettis of New Jersey. He has used running therapy with sixty patients between the ages of fifteen and fifty who were suffering from moderate depression and anxiety. He says he has obtained excellent results by using running in place of mood-altering drugs. Dr. Gettis sometimes runs with his patients and conducts a talk-therapy session as they jog along.

These results are consistent with what many people say they experience subjectively during and after physical activity. Exercise is a mood elevator. The very least that it does is keep one from dwelling on one's problems, serving as a kind of break from the cares of life. Having even a short depression-free interlude renews a person's hope that the illness itself will be limited. If it's possible to be free of it, even for a short time, maybe it isn't such a serious thing after all. And at best, exercise can produce long-term changes in mood and outlook.

Dr. David Pargman of Florida State University and others have shown that regular exercisers tend to be more emotionally stable, less likely to worry or become upset over minor frustrations, and suffer fewer minor psychosomatic disorders than nonexercisers.

A group of scientists at the School of Medicine of the University of California at Davis studied the effects of exercise on various risk factors for coronary heart disease, as well as on anxiety and depression. They studied a number of patients who had had heart disease and a number who had not; within each of these two groups some patients exercised and others didn't. After three sessions of exercise a week for twelve weeks, there were significant reductions in anxiety and depression among the people who exercised, whereas the people who did not exercise remained at the same level in all measures.

A group of psychiatrists and psychologists at the University of

Virginia noticed in their clinical practice that many of their depressed
patients derived benefits for long periods from regular physical exercise, and decided to study systematically the effects of exercise. They
did two studies, one with 167 subjects and another with 561 subjects,
all college students. They looked at a variety of activities, including
running (three days a week and five days a week), softball, wrestling,
and tennis. One group didn't take part in any exercise at all. The
researchers found that the groups who took part in regular exercise,
especially those who jogged five days a week for ten weeks, had the
greatest reduction in depression. The three-day-a-week jogging group,
the tennis group, and the wrestling and mixed exercise groups also
showed improvement. The group that played softball did not, however. The authors speculated that softball may not provide the sustained, rhythmic kind of activity most beneficial for depression.
Furthermore, the competition involved may prevent improvement,
because people tend to get depressed when they lose in competitive
events. The researchers suggested, therefore, that noncompetitive,
rhythmic activities are probably most effective. They also found that
exercise reduced anger and hostility, fatigue, tension and anxiety, and
that it increased cheerfulness, energy and general activity level. On the
basis of this study of over 700 subjects (including many who were not
depressed, as well as a number with recognized clinical depression),
the researchers concluded that any rational, safe and effective treatment regimen for depression should include a prescription for vigorous exercise in order to bring about and maintain optimal
physiological and psychological functioning.

The authors of this study conclude further that physical fitness
seems to be associated with a feeling of well-being and reduced anxiety
and depression, regardless of age, and that for maximum psychological gains, competitive events should not be stressed. They mentioned,
too, that while physical exertion on the job may be physiologically
beneficial, recreational exercise appears to be more beneficial psychologically, because the individual feels that he is *choosing* to do it and
thus taking control of his own life. Finally, they pointed out that
physicians and psychologists who personally take part in a physical
fitness program can be especially effective, because they serve as role
models for their patients.

Exercise and Self-Confidence

Dorothy Harris of Pennsylvania State University has done some very interesting work on the relationship between physical activity and attitudes toward challenging situations. The first phase of her project compared the attitudes of active people with those of people who were inactive. In the second phase, she took half of the inactive people, put them into an activity program for a year, and found that their attitudes toward activity changed in significant ways. For example, after a year of exercise, they were less likely to say they preferred to exercise by themselves, and now felt more comfortable exercising with others. They were also more likely to agree with the statements "I like games in which stamina and endurance are of importance" and "I play because I like the challenge created by play." One of the most marked changes was in response to this statement: "Each time I play I am reassured of my capacity to face physically demanding situations." All of the changes involved increased feelings of control and potency.

Our Own Fitness Can Help Others

Improvement in our psychological and physiological functioning can be important to those around us as well as to ourselves. The better we're feeling, mentally and physically, the more capable we'll be of helping other people with physical tasks or emotional support. Thomas Collingwood, a psychologist with the Dallas Police Department, believes that the counselor, who is helping other people to develop their physical, intellectual and emotional skills, has to be physically fit himself in order to be most effective.

Caring for yourself is an important part of caring for others. Women often feel that they must nurture others before taking care of themselves. Many men also work long hours in order to earn money and take care of their families, leaving little time to care for their own health. You have more than a right to take enough time to maintain your personal well-being—you have an *obligation* to do so in order to be most effective. You'll have the energy you need to be of service to others, and you'll serve in an ungrudging way because you know it's not being done *instead* of caring for your own well-being.

Besides, it's hardly fair to your family to hasten yourself along the path toward the degenerative diseases associated with a low-energy lifestyle, and possibly make yourself a burden to them. In the long as well as the short run, what's good for one member of the family is usually good for all the others.

Exerciser's High

In recent years a number of exercise scientists, clinicians and participants have wondered about the changes in the psychological state that often occur during or immediately following exercise. Because of the current popularity of running, much of the discussion and research has been centered around this form of exercise. However, the concepts can be applied to other activities similar to running in critical ways. For instance, the so-called runner's high, a feeling of euphoria that some runners experience, seems to come on after twenty to thirty minutes of relaxed running. The key factors are the rhythmic, continuous, moderately stimulating qualities of the activity; thus walking, cycling, swimming and cross-country skiing probably are just as likely to bring about this altered psychological state. In fact a recent study by Drs. Bonnie Berger and David Owen of Brooklyn College showed that after swimming people felt less tense, anxious, depressed and confused, and more vigorous, than before swimming. And dancing or exercising to music probably contributes to feelings of well-being by adding aesthetically pleasing sound.

Participants in sports like racquetball or basketball seldom report a high during the activity itself, but often do experience the feeling after stopping. The stop-and-go action of such sports probably interferes with the attainment of the calm and relaxed state required. On the other hand, psychiatrist Michael Sacks of Cornell Medical College points out that participants in any competitive sport frequently report a feeling of being "on" or "hot" when their minds and bodies are functioning at a peak level, and he suggests that this too is a form of high. It just may be easier for most people to get this good feeling in activities like running, swimming or walking because they require less skill.

The exerciser's high I'm referring to is not necessarily the same as the so-called altered state of consciousness some people experience during rhythmic exercise. Such an altered state is quite rare, and most exercisers don't experience it. I'm referring simply to a feeling of harmony with everything around you.

This enhanced psychological state may be due to the release of certain opiate-like chemicals in the brain during the exercise. These substances, called endorphins, have a chemical structure like that of morphine: they deaden pain and produce feelings of euphoria. Several recent studies have shown increased release of endorphins during exercise. Perhaps this is one aspect of the fight-or-flight response that is part of our evolutionary development. This idea is supported by studies done in Rome and Milwaukee, which showed that both moderate and strenuous exercise caused release of one of the key endorphins and the main stress hormone (ACTH) secreted by the pituitary gland.

However, a recent study at the University of Hawaii School of Medicine by Dr. Richard Markoff and colleagues casts doubt on the role of endorphins. They found improvement in several measures of mood following a normal day's run in a group of runners. However, the improved mood was not affected by the injection of a substance that blocks the effect of endorphins. This implies that the endorphins were not responsible for the mood changes.

Another chemical basis for the anti-depression effect of exercise concerns a group of neurotransmitters called amines, including norepinephrine, dopamine and serotonin. Depressed patients release less of these substances, and several treatments for depression (for example, anti-depressant medication and electroshock therapy) enhance the release of these amines at the connections between neurons in the brain (synapses). Exercise also seems to increase the synaptic release of these amines in depressed people.

It is unlikely that a one-to-one relationship exists between any one chemical event in the brain and a complex emotion in all kinds of people. Exercise elicits a complex range of physiological and neurological responses, and although the net result for most people is an improvement in mood, the effects are by no means uniform.

Whatever the neurological basis of the phenomenon, it's clear that many people experience pleasant feelings during and immediately after exercise. These feelings seem to occur most often when certain conditions exist. Conditions which seem conducive to the appearance of these feelings include:

1. Directing your attention inward.
2. Performing the exercise at a mildly stimulating, but not a stressful level.
3. Exercising in familiar surroundings.
4. Continuing the activity for at least twenty to thirty minutes.
5. Using some mental device to interfere with systematic thinking, such as concentrating on your breathing, counting, or repeating a favorite sound, phrase or prayer.
6. Imagining a pleasant scene, smell, or sound, one you associate with relaxation and pleasure.
7. Imagining your body functioning smoothly and effectively.

Some of these procedures are similar to those suggested earlier for eliciting the relaxation response. In fact, what you really want to do is elicit a kind of relaxation response while exercising, since relaxation is associated with an increase in alpha brain waves, which are in turn associated with feelings of extreme well-being. Herbert Benson and his colleagues at Harvard recently showed that it was possible to do just this, with the result that the energy needed to perform a standard amount of exercise on a stationary bicycle was reduced by about 10 percent.

Can You Become an Exercise Junkie?

As you might expect, people who are good at producing pleasant feelings in themselves when they exercise are inclined to spend a lot of time exercising. This has led some people to suggest that exercise can become an addiction. Psychiatrist William Glasser, the author of *Positive Addiction,* maintains that not all addictions are bad; those that are fulfilling and conducive to growth can be positive.

Most people would probably agree that a reasonable amount of daily exercise *is* a positive thing, physiologically and psychologically.

But what if it gets to a point where it takes precedence over your family and work? Dr. William Morgan has suggested that this situation can't be considered positive. But running guru George Sheehan disagrees. He argues that exercise *should* come before family and work. "First comes fitness and play, energy and self-discovery. We must first be made whole. Then we can return to the real world. We must first go back to being a child before we can do those adult things."

Certainly personal joy and fitness should be a high priority in everyone's life. But what if you reach a point where you are exercising several hours a day, hampering your ability to function adequately in other spheres of your life? It's possible with exercise, as with many other activities, to have too much of a good thing. But people who go this far are rare, and the possibility of becoming addicted to this degree is so unlikely that you needn't worry much about it. Being aware that the phenomenon does exist may be helpful: if you should get hooked on exercise, you won't let it progress to the point where you neglect other aspects of your life.

Exercise can't do everything. It can't alter all the factors in your life that may keep you from being happy. What it *can* do is make you better able to cope with them.

9

The High-Energy Diet

There are three main reasons for eating properly. The most obvious one is that you are what you eat. Your body builds and repairs itself from substances ingested in your food. Second, your ability to carry on your daily tasks requires you to transform energy in your food into the energy needed to keep your muscles and other organs functioning. If you are physically active, your needs for certain types of foods may be increased. Third, eating properly will help you lose weight or maintain a desirable weight while also maintaining your health and physical working capacity.

Let's start by discussing dietary guidelines for enhancement of health. Then we'll consider the type of diet that's appropriate for an active lifestyle and improvement of physical working capacity. Last, we'll look at caloric restriction for weight loss.

I. Nutrition for Optimal Health

The bulk of the food we eat is made up of proteins, fats and carbohydrates. These substances provide us with the energy we need to function, and are the building blocks for growth and repair of body tissues.

Some grasp of how they operate in the body is essential if you are going to make educated decisions about your nutrition.

Proteins

Proteins come from animal sources such as fish, poultry, lean meat, eggs, cheese, yogurt and milk, and plant sources such as cereals, bread, pasta, nuts and dried beans. Many of the body's structures— muscles, eyes, skin, hair—are made up of protein. The enzymes that regulate so many of the body's functions are proteins. And proteins help to form antibodies to fight infection. Although protein carries substantial numbers of calories, it appears to be used for energy metabolism mainly when the body runs low on carbohydrates and fats —that is, during starvation or severe dieting.

Protein is made up largely of amino acids, of which there are about twenty in animal tissue. The body is able to convert some amino acids into others, but there are eight essential amino acids that must be obtained from our diet. Protein from animal sources has an amino acid composition resembling that of human tissue, whereas protein from plant sources does not contain all the essential amino acids— though some vegetable proteins, such as those from rice and soybeans, are almost as complete as animal proteins. You can gain all the essential amino acids from plant sources by eating foods that are complementary. Some commonly eaten combinations (for example, milk with cereal, macaroni and cheese, peanut butter and bread, rice and beans) appear to be complementary.

One way to evaluate the protein content of food is to note the percent of the total energy the food provides that is protein. Some of the foods we normally think of as high in protein (e.g., lean beef) actually provide most of their energy in the form of fat (beef contains almost no carbohydrate). This is because fat contains more than twice as many usable calories per unit of weight as does protein or carbohydrate (9 calories per gram for fat and 4 calories per gram for protein and carbohydrate). Most forms of ground or prepared meats (e.g., hamburger, sausage, frankfurters, lunch meats) provide two-thirds or more of their energy in the form of fat. On the other hand, very lean fish (e.g., cod, haddock, halibut, sole, tuna in water, flounder) contain very little fat. Even fatty fish (e.g., herring, tuna in oil, salmon, sardines) are low in fat compared to meat.

Shellfish (e.g., lobsters, crayfish, scallops) and mollusks (oysters, mussels) are also high in protein and low in fat, and it now appears that shellfish are not so high in cholesterol as had previously been thought.

The proteins in an egg have the highest biological value for humans of all foods; since the egg is the complete food for the developing chick, it is naturally rich in essential nutrients. However, egg yolks contain very large amounts of cholesterol (whites do not), and when eaten in large numbers they raise blood cholesterol; thus they probably should not be utilized as a main source of protein.

Chicken is also high in protein and low in fat, *if the skin and the fat adhering to it are not eaten.* Without the skin, chicken provides about 66 percent of its calories in the form of protein, while with the skin, only about 33 percent of the calories are from protein and the rest are from fat.

The U.S. government recommends that protein make up no more than 8 to 10 percent of an adult's daily calorie intake. The World Health Organization recommends that your protein intake be about 7 percent of your total energy intake (about .57 grams per kilogram of weight). Since the average American adult gets about 12 percent of his calories from protein (and some studies say 15 to 17 percent), we're probably eating more protein than necessary.

Of course, pregnant and lactating women do need additional protein to provide for growth of the fetus and synthesis of milk protein. In the second half of pregnancy, the woman usually becomes quite sedentary and may gain weight without taking in many additional calories. In this case, the percentage of the intake that is protein should probably be at least 13 percent. If the woman remains normally active during pregnancy, as she should if there are no complications, then she will need to take in an additional 300 calories or so per day, and protein need not make up more than 12 percent. For the first six months or so of lactation, the woman needs about 500 extra calories, of which 80 should be protein. Her overall protein intake should be about 10 percent of total calories.

Since exercise stimulates protein synthesis in muscle, your protein needs will also increase a bit if you markedly increase your activity. If you are merely adding thirty to sixty minutes of exercise to an otherwise sedentary day, you may not need to increase your caloric intake, especially if you want to lose weight. In this case, check your diet to be sure your protein intake is sufficient to support the expected growth in muscle tissue. Ten percent of total calories should be plenty. If you increase your activity level markedly and you *don't* want to lose weight, you will naturally need to take in more total calories. By simply keeping the *percentage* of calories from protein at a constant level, you will be getting the increased protein you need for muscle growth.

During episodes of intense stress, infection or injury, protein requirements may be increased by as much as 100 percent. Intense physical exertion of the type seen in all-out competition may call forth hormonal changes similar to those seen in injury or infection. Thus the many adults now participating in competitive events such as marathons may need to increase their protein intakes for a week or so after the event.

Given all the scientific evidence and theory, what can we conclude as far as protein is concerned?

First, most Americans eat more protein than they need, especially in the form of animal protein, which frequently includes undesirable fat. Fish and skinless chicken are good animal protein sources, because they're low in fat.

Second, you can get plenty of protein from an exclusively vegetarian diet as long as a wide variety of grains, fruits, nuts, and vegetables is included. Including eggs and milk makes it even easier to get sufficient protein on a vegetarian diet. In fact, moving toward a more vegetarian diet may reduce your risk of heart disease.

Fat

Fats come from butter, margarine, salad oils, cooking oils, eggs, whole milk, cheese, ice cream, nuts, seeds, coconuts, palm, chocolates, avocados and meat.

The term *lipid* was invented by chemists to include all the chemical substances incorporated in what we know as fat, including triglycerides, cholesterol, and phospholipids. Although necessary for precise chemical work, for our purposes the distinction between the words *fat* and *lipid* is unimportant.

The main purpose of dietary fat is to provide a concentrated source of energy. Other purposes include aiding in the supply and absorption of fat-soluble vitamins (A, D, E, K); maintaining healthy skin; forming part of the structure of cell membranes; and serving as the precursors of prostaglandins, a class of hormonelike compounds that influence blood platelet function, smooth muscle contraction and other physiological functions.

Fat is extremely effective as an energy source because it carries a great number of calories per unit of weight compared to protein and carbohydrate. Fat is stored mainly as triglyceride in fat depots throughout the body. This tissue, known as adipose tissue, contains almost all fat and very little water. On the other hand, carbohydrate, the other main source of energy, is stored mainly as glycogen within muscle and liver cells with up to five times its weight in water. Birds must use fat almost exclusively for energy because if they stored much energy as carbohydrate they would be too heavy to fly. A typical adult man stores about 114,000 calories as fat and about 1,800 as glycogen and glucose (about 60 calories of glucose are carried in the blood). To gain an idea of the magnitude of this energy storage, remember that we use about 100 calories per mile of running. So all of the body's carbohydrate stores would be used up in 18 miles, whereas we could theoretically run 1,140 miles on our fat stores.

Another value of fat as an energy source is that during exercise it can be released from the fat depots into the blood and taken to any muscle which needs it. In contrast, once carbohydrate is stored in a muscle cell, it is only available as energy to that particular muscle cell, since the enzyme needed to break it down to glucose so it can be returned to the blood is not present in muscle cells. Thus one muscle used in a particular movement might be running out of glycogen while a neighboring muscle has more than enough.

Certain fatty acids must be present in the diet, since they are not synthesized in the body and do play important physiological roles, including reducing the tendency toward formation of blood clots and reducing blood cholesterol. These essential fatty acids are found in

Distribution of Fats in Common Foods

1. *High in polyunsaturated fats.*

   Safflower oil, corn oil, soft corn oil, certain margarines, walnuts, soybeans, sunflower seeds, sesame seeds, and oils made from these seeds.

2. *Moderately high in polyunsaturated fats.*

   Soybean oil, cottonseed oil, other soft margarines, commercial salad dressings, mayonnaise.

3. *High in monounsaturated fats.*

   Peanut oil, peanuts and peanut butter, olive oil, olives, almonds, pecans, cashews, brazil nuts, avocados.

4. *High in saturated fats.*

   Meats high in fat (e.g., sausages, cold cuts, prime cuts), chicken fat, meat drippings, lard, hydrogenated shortening, some stick margarines, coconut oil, butter and products with dairy fat (e.g., cheese, cream, whole milk, ice cream, chocolate, bakery items).

SOURCE: Adapted from *Nutrition and Health*, vol. 1, no. 1 (1979), M. Winick, "Diet and the Risk of Heart Attack."

polyunsaturated vegetable oils. (There are no known essential fatty acids in saturated fats.) Fats consisting mainly of saturated fatty acids are hard at room temperature, while those which are unsaturated or polyunsaturated are usually liquid. (The degree of saturation depends on the number of hydrogen atoms in the molecule; that's why saturated fats are called hydrogenated.) The table above shows which foods are high in which types of fat.

Animal fats tend to raise blood cholesterol, while unsaturated vegetable oils tend to lower it. The change is in the low-density lipoprotein (LDL) fraction, the one which is associated with coronary heart disease; the HDL (high-density lipoprotein) fraction doesn't seem to be affected by dietary change (with the exception of alcohol, as will be seen).

Cholesterol in the diet can also raise blood cholesterol levels and should be eaten in limited amounts only. In general, eating less satu-

Approximate Cholesterol Content in Milligrams of Selected Foods
(3-ounce portion, except for liquids)*

Beef	60
Chicken	51
Crabmeat	107
Fish fillet	60
Kidney	320
Lamb	60
Liver	256
Lobster	170
Mutton	55
Oysters	170
Pork	60
Shrimp	107
Veal	77
Milk Products	
Cheddar cheese	85
Cottage cheese	13
Cream cheese	102
Cheese spread	55
Ice cream	38
Whole milk (1 cup)	9
Skimmed milk (1 cup)	3

*Note that foods high in saturated fat are not necessarily high in cholesterol, though they may cause increases in blood cholesterol.
SOURCE: From values in *Composition of Foods,* U.S. Department of Agriculture Handbook No. 8, 1975.

rated fat will reduce your dietary cholesterol. Egg yolks are especially high in cholesterol: one egg contains about 250 milligrams of cholesterol, and the American Heart Association recommends a daily maximum of 300 milligrams. Foods from plant sources, such as vegetables, grains, fruits and margarine, contain no cholesterol. The table above gives the cholesterol content of some common foods.

The total fat in your diet shouldn't exceed 30 percent. Between 1900 and 1976 the average American increased the percent of his diet composed of fat from 32 to 42 percent, because of the increased availability of meat, eggs, and dairy products. This percentage is much too high for good health. However, fat makes an important contribution to our enjoyment of food, and if you go too far below 30 percent fat in your diet—if you follow Nathan Pritikin's recommendation to eat only 10 percent fat, for instance—you may find it an unrealistic and difficult regimen to maintain for the rest of your life.

Carbohydrates

Carbohydrates provide most of the energy in almost all human diets, except in those of highly developed, affluent societies. In the United States, about 46 percent of our calories come in the form of carbohydrate, while in very poor countries up to 90 percent of the diet may be from this source.

Carbohydrates are synthesized in green plants from water and carbon dioxide, with sunlight providing the extra energy stored in the carbohydrate formed. This energy is eventually released in all our energy-demanding physiological processes, including muscular contraction and maintenance of body temperature. The end products of the energy-releasing processes are carbon dioxide and water, which are returned to the environment so the plants can reuse them and continue the cycle. Of the carbohydrates in food, some can be digested and utilized by man (available carbohydrates), and some are composed of fiber, which is relatively indigestible (unavailable carbohydrates).

The simplest dietary sugar is glucose, the same glucose present in our blood. Very few natural foods, except a few fruits like grapes, contain much glucose. However, glucose is combined with fructose, a simple sugar found in honey and fruit, to make up sucrose, which is the table sugar in common use. Lactose is the main sugar found in milk. Of course, the sweet taste of sugar is why such large amounts are consumed in rich societies today. If the sweetness of sucrose is arbitrarily set at 100, the relative sweetness to our taste of fructose is 170, glucose 50 and lactose 20.

Starch is a complex carbohydrate made up of hundreds of glucose units strung together. Starch is then broken down to glucose again in our digestive tracts. Starch is found largely in potatoes and in cereal grains such as wheat, rice, corn, oats, barley, and rye.

The key change in the diets of Americans in this century has been a marked reduction in starch intake. Fat intake has risen about 25 percent and total carbohydrate intake has dropped about 25 percent; protein intake has remained fairly stable. Of the carbohydrates, a dramatic shift from complex to simple has occurred. From 1889 to 1961, our yearly intake of cereal products dropped from 358 pounds per person to 146, a decrease of 59 percent. At the same time our yearly intake of sugars and syrups went from 53 to 115 pounds per person, a rise of 117 percent. This shift from dietary starch to sugar has probably contributed to the increased incidence of diabetes and CHD.

One of the key differences between complex and simple carbohydrates is the amount of fiber in them, and one result of this shift to simple carbohydrates has been a precipitous drop in dietary fiber intake.

Different types of dietary fiber have somewhat different physiological effects, and much is still unknown about the mechanisms through which fiber influences health. In general, fiber binds water, thereby increasing fecal weight and shortening the transit time of fecal matter through the colon. This relieves constipation and colonic pressure during defecation, thereby perhaps preventing hemorrhoids, varicose veins, and diverticulitis. The lower incidence of colon and rectal cancer in the countries where high-fiber diets are eaten may be due to the shorter time that the feces stay in the colon and their increased water content; if any carcinogens are present in the fecal matter, the colon walls are exposed to it for a shorter time and in a lower concentration.

So what can we conclude about the role of carbohydrate in the diet? Certainly, we tend to eat too much simple carbohydrate, mainly in the form of refined sucrose. Sucrose is energy-rich and nutrient-poor. It also contributes to dental caries. About 70 percent of the sucrose we eat is consumed in processed foods and soft drinks, so we do not see it. It is added to many foods to enhance their flavor and encourage you to buy them rather than the brand next to them on the supermarket shelf.

Fruits and fruit juices also contain simple sugars, so they can satisfy our appetite for sweets to a large extent. Modern agriculture and transportation make fruit available to us throughout the year, which makes many nutrients and fibers available all year round.

Carbohydrates should be the mainstay of your diet, in the form of a variety of whole grains, fruits, and vegetables. A sudden switch to a high-fiber diet can lead to abdominal discomfort, flatulence and frequent defecation; there is a great deal of individual variation in how much fiber can be eaten comfortably. So change your diet gradually so that you can monitor your physiological responses and allow your body to adjust to the change.

And how can you tell if you are getting enough fiber? One rather gross technique is to observe whether your stools tend to sink or float. Soft and large stools will tend to float. You should also find that your bowel movements are more comfortable due to less straining, and perhaps more frequent as well.

Alcohol

Alcohol is another energy carrier, and some people take in significant amounts of calories in the form of beer, wine, and spirits. For example, if two people share a liter carafe of wine with dinner, each would be taking in about 350 calories, or about 25 percent of the calories used in one day by basic physiological processes. Beer has about 250 to 300 calories per liter and 80 proof spirits (e.g., brandy, rum, gin, and whiskey) have about 65 calories in a typical one-ounce shot. So to the extent that you include alcohol in your diet, you need to cut back somewhat on other foodstuffs.

For the most part, beer, wine, and spirits contain empty calories in that they contain very few vitamins and minerals. Thus if alcohol constitutes too large a proportion of your diet, you may become malnourished.

Ingested alcohol is absorbed into the blood very quickly from the stomach and small intestine. Food in the stomach slows the rate of absorption, and more concentrated spirits will produce higher peak blood levels of alcohol than mixed drinks, beer or wine. Due to differing body size and other factors, people vary a great deal in how much alcohol will produce relaxation, a "glow" or signs of drunkenness, so you need to become sensitive to your own responses and adjust your own intake accordingly.

The damaging effects of alcohol abuse are well known. Most fatal auto accidents are probably associated with excessive drinking, and alcoholism is a serious medical and social problem. Many people do not realize, however, that moderate drinking has beneficial consequences for health.

A number of studies have shown that moderate drinkers are likely to live longer and have fewer heart attacks than either teetotalers or those who drink excessively. The physiological mechanisms for this relationship are unclear. One possibility has to do with high-density lipoproteins. Moderate alcohol intake elevates HDL, and high HDL is associated with a reduced risk of heart disease. A study at the Bowman-Gray School of Medicine of Wake Forest University showed that in monkeys the inclusion of alcohol in the diet retarded the atherosclerosis produced by a high-cholesterol diet, probably because the alcohol raised the HDL and altered the structure of the LDL molecules. Another possibility is that the relaxing effect of alcohol reduces blood pressure, which in turn reduces the risk of heart disease. Some studies in a home for the aged showed that serving beer and wine with meals improved social interaction, lessened the incidence of physical problems, and reduced prescriptions of psychotropic drugs.

The levels of alcohol intake that appear to be associated with improved health are fairly substantial—as much as 56 grams of alcohol per day. This represents about 6 ounces of 80 proof spirits, 20 ounces of table wine, or four and a half 12-ounce bottles of beer. This amount seems to be well within the safe limits for health, especially when accompanied by nutritionally adequate food (though many nutritionists are afraid to recommend any amount of alcohol at all, despite what the data show). Damage to the liver seems to occur in many people when consumption reaches a daily level of 100 to 150 grams.

Some nutritionists believe that subtle and eventually serious damage to the liver, heart and gastrointestinal system may result from long-term ingestion of more than one to two drinks a day, which comes to about half of the 56 grams many researchers consider safe.

The 56 grams mentioned above is probably a *safe upper level for any given day.* Drinking up a week's allotment on the weekend is probably not safe. Researchers at the Medical College of Wisconsin found that binge drinkers had significantly higher levels of blood-vessel blockage than those who drank regularly and moderately. In addition, the intoxication that usually results from binge drinking certainly increases the risk of accidents. And the liver may also be put under some strain to metabolize such large amounts.

There is considerable controversy in medical circles over the question of whether a pregnant woman should drink at all, due to possible effects on the fetus. The National Institute on Alcohol Abuse and Alcoholism suggests that a woman may reach risk level at two to six drinks a day, and it may be prudent to have no more than one drink a day during pregnancy.

Other Nutrients

In addition to the energy carriers, our diets include a variety of substances that regulate our physiological processes, including water, minerals, vitamins, and trace elements. Though we know a great deal about nutrition, there is much more that we don't yet know. If we had complete information on all essential nutrients and were able to package them in a pill, we could theoretically dispense with food. At present, the surest and most enjoyable way to obtain the nutrients we need is to eat a wide variety of natural foods. Those who want a thorough, intelligent outline of what is currently known about human nutrition are advised to read *Jane Brody's Nutrition Book.*

A Healthful Diet

For the most part, it seems sensible to move in the direction of the recommendations that came out of the 1977 U.S. Senate report on nutrition and human needs (see the table opposite for a synopsis), though these recommendations may not go far enough. The Senate committee interviewed many nutritional scientists and did an excellent job of sifting the evidence, although some nutritionists argue that the committee moderated their recommendations too much because of pressure from the dairy and meat industries.

Recommended Diet
(*percentages of total intake*)

	Current U.S. Diet	U.S. Senate Committee Dietary Goals	High-Energy Lifestyle Diet
Fat	42	30	25
Saturated	16	10	10
Mono- and Polyunsaturated	26	20	15
Protein	12	12	10
Carbohydrate	46	58	65
Complex and Naturally Occurring Sugars	28	48	55
Refined and Processed Sugars	18	10	10

The bulk of your diet should be in the form of complex carbohydrates and naturally occurring sugars.* The Senate Committee recommends 48 percent of intake in this category, with another 10 percent in the form of refined and processed sugars, for a total carbohydrate intake of about 58 percent carbohydrate. The current American diet includes about 28 percent complex carbohydrates and natural sugars, and 18 percent refined sugars.

Strive for 55 percent complex carbohydrate and natural sugars, and less than 10 percent refined sugars, for a total carbohydrate intake of about 65 percent. You may not be able to eliminate refined sugars altogether unless you live a very ascetic life. Most people like to eat sweets once in a while.

My recommendations are based partly on the idea that you will adopt a high-energy lifestyle that will require you to eat about 500 calories per day more than the average person that the Senate Committee was considering. Since the extra energy required should be in a form most effective in supporting this type of active lifestyle, it should be largely carbohydrate. Thus, even though the *percent* of your

---

*For a breakdown of the percentage of total calories in the form of fats, proteins and carbohydrates in certain foods, see the Appendix (page 186)

diet which is made up of fat and protein will decline, the *total amount* of these nutrients that you ingest will be slightly greater than that proposed by the committee. The extra carbohydrate should come almost entirely from fruits, vegetables, whole-grain breads and cereals, rice, pasta and potatoes, which will assure a substantial amount of natural fiber.

One myth that must be laid to rest is that bread is unhealthy and to be avoided, especially in weight control. This idea leads some people to eat hamburgers while not eating the bun. *If a choice has to be made you are probably better off with the bun than the burger,* since the burger provides most of the calories in the form of saturated fat, and is much more calorically dense than the bun.

The committee recommends that fat consumption be dropped from the current level of about 40 percent to 30 percent, while protein intake should remain at about 12 percent. It seems to me that the fat intake should be somewhat lower, about 25 percent, while I agree with the committee's suggestion that more should be in the form of unsaturated fat and less in saturated fat, perhaps 15 and 10 percent respectively. The protein percentage should drop slightly to about 10 percent, but remain about the same in amount, as you adopt a high-energy lifestyle and increase your total intake. Increases in exercise do not appear to require increases in protein intake. As you reduce your saturated fat intake, your intake of cholesterol will also drop.

I concur with the Senate committee recommendation that salt consumption be reduced markedly, by 50 to 60 percent. You will need to reduce your consumption of presalted foods as well as reduce the salt used in cooking and seasoning. Try using other seasonings, such as pepper and other spices, garlic, onion, vinegar and lemon juice. Cooking with fruit (e.g., pineapples, oranges) or fruit juices can also reduce the need for salt.

I do not recommend that you take any supplementary vitamins or minerals on a regular basis. Eating a large volume and a wide variety of nutritious foods is the surest way to get enough of the essential nutrients. Relying on pills for almost magical qualities is contrary to my intuition as well as being as yet unsupported by scientific research.

Of course these recommendations are very general and may not apply to you at any particular time. For example, during pregnancy and lactation, many of your body's needs change dramatically. Always work with your personal physician to decide what specific action you should take.

Suggestions for Meals

If you adopt these recommendations, what will a typical day's intake look like?

For breakfast, you'll eat citrus fruits and/or juices (and perhaps other fruit as well); whole-grain breads with cottage cheese, unsweetened peanut butter, or a little butter or margarine; cereal with nonfat or low-fat milk; and perhaps a cup of tea or coffee with low-fat milk, if you like, but without sugar. Having fruit with bread or cereal can provide a delicious taste and reduce your need for butter or jelly. Two or three times a week, have an egg, preferably poached or boiled rather than fried, and served with bread. Many people don't feel like eating much in the morning, but gradually increase the amount you eat at breakfast until it approaches at least a quarter of your daily calories. This meal follows many hours of fasting, and your body needs energy for the active life you'll be leading. If you're watching your weight, it's especially important to avoid feeling so hungry by lunch and dinner that you overeat before you even notice it. Try adding things you don't ordinarily think of as breakfast food: a grilled cheese sandwich, grilled tomatoes, brown rice with leftover vegetables or nuts and raisins.

If you feel the need for a between-meal snack, have some fruit. It satisfies the sweet tooth and is quite filling, making it an excellent dessert as well.

For lunch you might have a sandwich or two made up of whole grain bread filled with such things as tuna, sliced turkey roll, low-fat cheese, lettuce and tomato. Or have a vegetable plate or a fresh vegetable salad or a fruit salad with cottage cheese.

For dinner, you might eat a small serving of lean meat or fish, starch (potato, rice, pasta), vegetables, bread and salad. As you go along you can gradually reduce the amount of meat or fish and increase the amount of the other ingredients until you think of the meat and fish as condiments rather than aliments. Such a change in attitude will greatly facilitate an increase in complex carbohydrates and decrease in saturated fat and animal protein. You might dispense with meat altogether for a few dinners a week, especially if you had some for lunch. Main dishes that include complementary proteins, cheese or eggs can assure an adequate supply of essential amino acids.

For a beverage with meals, drink water, although wine might enhance the festive aura of dinner. Two or three cups of tea and perhaps coffee each day are probably okay, especially if they are not too strong. If you want to avoid caffeine, you might try herb tea, decaffeinated coffee, or a coffee substitute.

For dessert or snack a few times a week, you might have cake, pie, cookies, ice cream or pudding. One of the beauties of a high-energy lifestyle is that you can eat more food, including some delicious desserts. Of course, do not overdo it, or let these kinds of foods crowd out the more nutritious ones.

Dining out can be a problem, since foods rich in fat and sugar are very tempting. Fortunately, the increasing health consciousness of Americans is leading restaurants to offer lighter foods, salad bars and so on. Watch out for words on the menu such as *buttery, sauteed, fried, creamed, au gratin, cheese sauce, à la mode, en casserole, prime, hash, pot pie,* and *hollandaise.* On the other hand, look for descriptions that include words such as *pickled, tomato sauce, steamed, in broth, poached, garden fresh, roasted, stir-fried* and *cocktail sauce.* Seek out restaurants specializing in fish, salads, breads, fruits and vegetables rather than those emphasizing steaks, chops and rich desserts.

Pay attention to what you eat. Many people become so accustomed to eating large amounts of junk food, potato chips, cookies and so on, that they don't even notice (or really enjoy) it. If you are careful about what you eat, you will find that a healthy diet can provide enormous pleasure along with the satisfaction of knowing that you are contributing to your health and well-being.

II. Food for Sport

Protein

For many years it was believed that people who used their muscles in strenuous exercise needed to eat large amounts of meat to replenish in some way the protein used up in the exercise.

In the past thirty years or so, scientific studies have shown that protein does not play a major role in the release of energy during exercise, except in cases where insufficient fat and carbohydrate are available, as in starvation. Fairly small amounts of dietary protein are sufficient to support the tissue building and repairing functions for which protein is necessary.

The Importance of Carbohydrate

As long ago as 1939, two Scandinavian physiologists, E. H. Christensen and O. Hansen, showed that men could run for about 4 hours after several days on a diet high in carbohydrates, but could run at the same pace for only about 1.5 hours after eating a high-fat diet, and 2 hours after a normal mixed diet, before becoming exhausted. They also showed that the runners eating the high-carbohydrate diet released most of the energy from carbohydrate, whereas those eating the high-fat diet released most of the energy from fat. Subsequent studies have shown that a high-carbohydrate diet increases storage of glycogen in the muscles and liver, and that the depletion of this carbohydrate is often associated with exhaustion during marathon endurance tasks.

These studies led to the procedure called carbohydrate loading or packing, which is designed to bring the body's stores of glycogen up to maximal levels on the day of a marathon. The procedure begins seven days before the event. For three days (called the depletion phase) you engage in long workouts designed to deplete the glycogen stores. On these days you eat a diet almost devoid of carbohydrate (e.g., eggs, fish, meat) to assure the most complete depletion possible, in order to turn on the enzyme which increases synthesis of glycogen. For the next three days you reduce your exercise to a minimum and eat a diet extremely high in carbohydrate, which will now be stored with greater efficiency. This is called the repletion or loading phase. On the seventh day, instead of resting, you presumably go out and win. Many distance runners now use this type of procedure and report up to a ten-minute improvement in marathon time as a result.

However, there are a number of reasons to doubt the wisdom of this procedure, especially of the depletion phase. In the absence of carbohydrate for fuel, as occurs during the depletion phase, the body burns fat, leading to the accumulation in the blood of ketone bodies, a product of fat metabolism. In large amounts, this leads to ketosis, which may result in kidney damage, irritability and depression. Low blood glucose and feelings of extreme fatigue may also result. In fact, a recent study by Dr. David Costill and colleagues showed that glycogen loading was just as effective if a diet with 40 percent carbohydrate was used for the first three days of the regimen.

Some rare but potentially serious problems can also arise during the repletion phase, including:

1. electrocardiographic abnormalities and chest pain.

2. swelling of the prostate gland and painful urination due to inadequate fluid intake (since glycogen storage requires large amounts of water, you should drink at least eight glasses a day).

3. potassium deficiency (this can be avoided by eating fruits high in potassium).

4. release from the muscles of myoglobin, a large protein, which may damage the kidney.

A minor problem, but one worth knowing about, is that you will probably gain a few pounds due to the extra water stored along with the glycogen. At the start of the race, this extra weight seems to be a handicap, but it comes in handy as the race progresses and you lose water in sweat. As the stored glycogen is utilized for energy release, the water stored with it becomes available to the circulation and slows the rate of dehydration.

Any radical procedure may have radical consequences for the body. Perhaps carbohydrate loading will enhance your marathon endurance, but it *may* also cause permanent damage. And this procedure is so new that the long-range effects of repeatedly undergoing it are unknown. For these reasons, you might be better off simply reducing the number and length of your workouts and increasing your carbohydrate intake for the last few days before a big event.

Marathon running is not the only type of event that falls into the class of marathon endurance, although running is an easy sport with which to experiment. In fact, Dr. Bengt Saltin, the distinguished Scandinavian physiologist, showed with motion pictures that soccer players who followed the carbohydrate loading procedure exhibited less evidence of fatigue in the second half of the game than those who did not load. Any sport that demands a high level of energy expenditure for upwards of thirty to sixty minutes is probably influenced by glycogen storage.

Of course, most of us are not so interested in getting ready for events which require all-out effort as we are in carrying on our routine recreational activities effectively. Simply eating the diet which is recommended for optimal health will generally provide sufficient amounts of all essential nutrients.

Eating, Drinking and Exercising

What should you eat and drink before, during and after a workout or event? In this area, there are also a number of old myths that have been exploded by scientific investigation.

One myth involves how much time should be allowed to pass between eating and subsequent exercise. True, *strenuous* exercise demands that blood be diverted from the digestive system so that oxygen can be brought to the working muscles, thereby interfering with digestion, and possibly leading to a cramp or stitch. However, during light and moderate exercise there is sufficient blood to support both the needed oxygen transport and digestive processes. Moreover, the general increase in circulation and metabolism elicited by mild exercise seems to facilitate the clearance of newly digested fats from the blood. Thus a *leisurely* walk after a heavy meal helps to metabolize some of the fat that is being digested before it has a chance to be stored in your fat cells, or even in the cells of your coronary arteries. However, you should allow at least two to three hours to elapse after eating before a *strenuous* workout.

Special caution must be observed before a competitive event due to the emotional factors involved. Part of the fight-or-flight response involves a shutdown of digestive processes. For this reason many competitors find it hard to digest their food on the day of a contest. Use your own experience as a guide, but generally a pregame meal should be eaten at least three to five hours prior to the event, and should consist of easily digested foods that are low in fat and high in carbohydrate (but without too much fiber). Some examples are orange juice, toast with honey rather than butter, pancakes with very little butter, and tea or coffee. Don't eat any simple sugars less than two hours before an event, since they are quickly absorbed into the bloodstream and their rate of absorption is the trigger for the release of insulin. In an hour or so the blood glucose level is lower than normal, a phenomenon called rebound hypoglycemia, and you might have to go through the whole event in a hypoglycemic state. Pancake syrup, molasses and honey contain simple sugars and should be taken in moderation. Breads, pasta (spaghetti and macaroni), rice and potatoes are high in complex carbohydrate and are digested more slowly, thereby stimulating insulin to be released more gradually. Fruits contain fructose, which is also a simple sugar, but for some as-yet-unexplained reason, it seems to be absorbed by the digestive system somewhat more slowly, and is therefore preferable to refined sugar. Furthermore, fruit contains many important nutrients often lost when sugar is refined.

Many athletes now take a cup or two of tea or coffee about an hour before a marathon endurance event because the caffeine in these drinks cause fatty acids to be released into the blood. The muscles then use the fat for energy to a greater extent and the muscle glycogen is not used up so quickly, thereby improving performance.

One essential but often overlooked constituent of the active person's diet is water, a vital part of the body's temperature-regulating apparatus. Most of the energy liberated by the body is in the form of heat; only about 20 percent ends up in the form of actual mechanical work done. Most of this heat must be removed from the body to avoid dangerous increases in body temperature. During vigorous exercise the amount of heat generated is so great that we must rely largely on the formation and vaporization of sweat. Evaporation is a process that uses up large amounts of heat. Without it we would find our body temperature rising to dangerous levels very quickly during exercise.

As an extreme example, marathon runners may have sweat losses of six pounds per hour for two to three hours. Even though they drink quite a bit during the run to replace some of the sweat loss, they may lose ten pounds of body weight, which corresponds to about five quarts or 12 percent of total body water, during the run. Athletes in some sports report weight losses up to as much as seventeen pounds in a game or practice session.

Most of the weight loss is water, and most of that comes from the blood plasma. A loss of as little as 2 percent of body weight by exercise-induced sweating can compromise the ability of the cardio-vascular system to supply blood to both working muscles and skin. The reduction of blood volume means less blood returns to the heart and less is pumped out with each beat. The heart tries to compensate by beating faster. A higher heart rate indicates a greater myocardial oxygen consumption—that is, a greater cardiac strain. Therefore, anyone who needs to keep his heart rate below some given point due to heart disease must be especially careful not to incur large and unreplaced sweat losses.

Even if your heart is healthy and capable of vigorous effort and you are not concerned with the cardiac strain involved, the loss of blood plasma can lead to reduced blood pressure, dizziness and collapse, and dangerously high body temperatures. Consequently, water balance is one of the most important matters in all of sports medicine and exercise physiology.

So drink a lot of water before, during and after any event or practice that lasts longer than an hour or so. And don't rely exclusively on your thirst as a guide, since people only drink about half as much as they lose in sweat. Consciously drink more than you feel like drinking, especially if the air temperature is high and you are sweating pro-fusely. Take many small drinks instead of a few large ones, since a large amount in the stomach at one time can hinder the movement of the diaphragm and feel quite uncomfortable.

The water should be cold, since some heat is absorbed from the body just to warm the water to body temperature. Moreover, cool fluids are emptied from the stomach into the blood more rapidly than warm fluids. Many people worry that cold drinks will cause stomach cramps, but this fear seems to be groundless; gastric distress is related more to how much you drink than to the temperature of the drink.

One practice you might make a habit of is starting any extended period of exercise by taking a cup or so of fluid within ten minutes of beginning. Undoubtedly you empty your bladder before exercising so that you don't have to worry about needing to urinate in the middle of your exercise, but liquid drunk within about ten minutes of starting does not have time to pass through your kidneys and reach your bladder before you start. Once you do start, most of the blood pumped by your heart will be diverted to the working muscles, very little will go to your kidneys and almost no urine will be formed.

Is Salt Replacement Necessary?

Since sweat tastes salty, we realize that we are losing salt as well as water, leading to the misconception that it is urgent to replace this salt during or immediately after the exercise. Small amounts of potassium, calcium and magnesium are also lost in sweat, but so little of these substances are lost that there is little need to be concerned about their replacement.

As salty as sweat tastes, it's less salty than body fluids, so you are losing proportionately more water than salt. Thus when you sweat profusely, the *concentration* of the salt and other minerals left behind in the body *increases* even though the total amount has decreased, and after the exercise the normal concentrations need to be regained. So the main requirement the body has is for replacement of *water* rather than salt. You can lose up to about six pounds (three quarts) of water without needing salt tablets; simply salting slightly more heavily at your next meal should suffice for salt replacement. If the exercise is so prolonged, as in all-day hiking or cross-country skiing, that even more than six pounds of water is lost and replaced, some attention should be paid to salt replacement. Most of the commercial sport drinks available include salt and other minerals lost in sweat. Or add some salt to the water you carry in a canteen (a seven-grain salt tablet per pint should be adequate). Make sure the salt concentration is low enough for the water to be palatable.

Can Glucose Improve Performance?

Another ingredient often included in athletic drinks is sugar. This makes some sense in light of the importance of carbohydrate to endurance performance. However, drinks containing a high concentration of solids in the form of salt and sugar are emptied from the stomach much more slowly than plain water. Thus if the main purpose of fluid ingestion is to get water back into the blood plasma quickly, consumption of a strong sugar drink is a poor way to do it. Only in events classified as marathon endurance events is it necessary to worry about carbohydrate depletion at all. In this case, a mild sugar drink of less than 2.5 percent sugar (for example, one ounce per quart of water or 25 grams per liter) can be useful in replacing water while providing valuable energy. This type of drink can be emptied quickly from the stomach, thereby supplying the water and sugar to the body rapidly. The sugar will be absorbed and ready for use by the muscles in about five to seven minutes. Taking in sugar *during* an event does not cause rebound hypoglycemia, as it does with ingestion twenty minutes to two hours *before* the exercise, because the exercise itself suppresses the insulin response.

In general, carbonated soft drinks and the commercial athletic drinks available are not the best beverages to drink. They usually have too much sugar in them to permit fast emptying of the stomach. And the athletic drinks that include many of the minerals lost in sweat are somewhat unpalatable, thereby reducing your motivation to drink them and subverting the primary goal of water replacement. Diluting these drinks with two or three parts water overcomes these problems. Fruit juices must be similarly diluted because they are rather high in solids, which hold water in the stomach. These are probably the best replacement drinks because they are real foods.

Tasks in Which Water Is Not Critical

Up to now, we've focused on conditions where large amounts of sweat are formed and water is the most important ingredient to be replaced. But if you hike, ski, or engage in any other activity that is carried on for several hours, especially in cold weather where evaporation is not the main mechanism of heat loss, carbohydrate may be the substance most in need of replacement. In this case, small quantities of a sugar solution containing as much as 10 ounces of sugar per quart of water (about 250 grams per liter) will be released slowly from the stomach and provide a steady source of energy for the working muscles. Fruits with high sugar concentrations (for example, raisins, dried apricots) and of course candy bars can also provide quick energy.

When the relative humidity is low, you may sweat quite a bit and not notice it because it evaporates so quickly. So you should probably replace some fluids any time you exercise for more than an hour or two, regardless of how much (or little) you seem to be sweating.

How to Speed the Recovery Processes

And what is the best way to help the body to recover from the stress it has been experiencing? Plenty of minerals and carbohydrates are called for, and beer seems to be the predominant choice of many athletes. But fruit juices are more desirable because they are more complete foods than beer. Furthermore, strenuous exercise is inherently relaxing, so you probably do not need the additional relaxation provided by the alcohol in the beer. You may find yourself crossing that thin line between relaxation and sleep!

Fruit juices and fruits in general, especially bananas, also contain potassium, one of the minerals lost in sweat. Large losses of potassium can upset the mineral balance in the body, and some authorities have suggested that large-scale replacement of this mineral is necessary. Animal studies have shown that a low-potassium diet can severely impair endurance capacity and also greatly increase the risk of heatstroke. However, Dr. David Costill and his colleagues at Ball State University found that even when subjects did dehydrating endurance exercise on four successive days and ate a diet extremely low in potassium, they were able to maintain muscle and plasma potassium at normal levels. Still, the seriousness of the consequences of heatstroke suggest that we eat plenty of fruit, which is good for general health anyway.

Becoming Your Own Sports Nutritionist

The question of what to eat and drink to support an active lifestyle is a complex one, and no one prescription will be appropriate for all people under all environmental conditions and for all kinds of exercise. Therefore, you should make an attempt to understand the underlying physiology so you can in a sense become your own coach and nutritionist. Only you can integrate your own bodily sensations with scientifically derived guidelines to formulate a personal nutritional plan.

III. Eating for Weight Control

Although the switch from a low-energy to a high-energy lifestyle is the basis for permanent weight control, the composition of the diet is also quite important, because an active life can be most effectively pursued if the diet is full of appropriate nutrients as well as calories. Eating large amounts of empty calories in the form of sugar will not do.

If you want to count calories, see the Appendix for a table that gives the number of calories in many common foods. For a more complete list, write the U.S. Superintendent of Documents, Washington, D.C. 20402 for the handbook *Composition of Foods.* Any number of diet books go into calorie-counting in some detail, but calorie-counting encourages people to think of food in a negative way, and it is hardly a permanent lifestyle change.

A better approach is to use a system of food exchanges, as described in a number of sources, including *Jane Brody's Nutrition Book.* This system allows you to choose a variety of foods to make up a changing daily menu of a certain number of calories. The calories in the portions have all been determined by the Institute of Human Nutrition at Columbia University.

Even the food-exchange approach requires that you govern your intake quite precisely. You might want to adopt a less precise approach, which may lead to a somewhat slower weight loss, but which is probably the best long-term strategy because it involves a gradual and permanent change in eating habits. Simply shift your diet in the direction advocated in this book: that is, toward a high-carbohydrate and low-fat intake, with more of the protein coming from vegetables and grains than from meat and dairy products. Cut down on fat even more than recommended earlier, and avoid empty calories such as alcohol and sugar. Keep careful track of your weight on a daily basis, and aim for a one-pound weight loss per week by simply eating smaller portions of everything. As you approach the desired weight, you can add more food to the diet. Many people find that wine with dinner, even though it provides some empty calories, enables them to enjoy and savor a meal including less food than they're used to.

By eating more bread and vegetables, instead of meat which has so much calorically dense fat in it, the *volume* of food eaten may be maintained, along with the length of the mealtime. The dinner table is an important social setting, and a diet that allows a person to participate normally is more likely to be followed permanently than one that requires eating patterns radically different from those of the rest of the family.

The table opposite provides lists of foods to be avoided and those which are desirable on a reducing diet.

If you've decided you want to include caloric restriction as part of your weight-loss program, but find it difficult to change your eating habits, try using some of the same behavior-modification techniques talked about in connection with exercise (page 40–43). Read them again and see how many of them you can adapt to your eating behaviors. For instance, set small, specific and easily attainable goals for yourself. Be flexible, changing your goals if you find they're unrealistic or impossible for you to live with. Keep a diary of your daily eating, just as you do of your daily physical activity. Work with someone else. Reward yourself for each small success. Here are some more suggestions:

1. In order to avoid impulse buying of foods that don't fit into your evolving diet and changing lifestyle, (a) make a shopping list before going out and purchase only what's on the list; (b) shop after a good meal; (c) shop with a friend who is also trying to switch to a high-carbohydrate, low-fat diet.

Foods to Be Avoided or Encouraged on a Weight-Loss Diet

To be avoided: sugar, candies, chocolate, jams, jellies, honey, syrup, molasses, canned or frozen fruits preserved with sugar, dried fruits, cakes, pastries, puddings, ice cream, whole milk, cream, peas, sweet corn, lima and navy beans, lentils, nuts, salad dressings, mayonnaise, cream sauces, fatty meats or fishes, sausages, fried foods, sweetened fruit juices, carbonated beverages, all alcoholic drinks.

To be taken as desired: vegetables such as asparagus, eggplant, string beans, broccoli, brussels sprouts, cabbage, cauliflower, celery, cucumber, leeks, lettuce, mushrooms, onion, parsley, peppers, pumpkin, radishes, sauerkraut, spinach, squash, tomatoes, turnips; drinks such as water, tea, coffee, sugar-free fruit drinks, sugar-free carbonated drinks; saccharin preparations; spices such as pepper, vinegar, mustard, herbs, pickles, relish, soy sauce; unthickened gravy.

2. When eating out, avoid restaurants specializing in high-fat foods and seek out those emphasizing salads, vegetables and fish. For a breakdown of the nutritional composition of some fast foods, see the Appendix (page 184).

3. Avoid starving yourself early in the day so that you feel justified in stuffing yourself at dinner and later. Spread your calories fairly evenly throughout the day. People who eat all their daily calories in one or two large meals become fatter than people who space the same number of calories over four to six meals a day.

4. Avoid nibbling at nearby foods that you really don't want or need. Don't leave extra food on the table; dish out as much as you want and put the rest away before starting to eat. At parties, stay away from all those tempting finger foods, or decide in advance how many you'll have and stick to it.

5. Sometimes we eat inappropriately when we're tense, angry or bored; we have learned to use eating as a way to give ourselves pleasure at such times. So use alternative activities when you get these feelings. For example, go for a walk, do some calisthenics, sit down and elicit the relaxation response, or take a hot bath. In other

words, break the connection between inappropriate eating and these feelings by finding other ways to stimulate, relax and please yourself.

6. Whenever you make an appropriate food choice or substitute a different activity, you can reinforce the behavior by thinking of yourself as strong, in charge of your own life. You can also use some of the imaging techniques I mentioned in connection with exercise. For example, imagine yourself svelte and fit in a bathing suit.

If you also increase your routine walking and specific aerobic exercise sessions, in addition to reducing your caloric intake, you may be able to achieve an energy deficit of about 1,000 calories a day. This adds up to 7,000 calories per week and should lead to a fat loss of about two pounds per week. Some additional water loss will also result in the first week or two, since the total carbohydrate ingested will probably fall somewhat.

As you approach your goal weight you will be tempted to stop the diet and resume a more normal diet, including substantial amounts of complex carbohydrate. This may lead to a retention of some water and gain in weight. If so, don't panic. The water goes into the lean tissue of the body; it is not making you "fatter." In order to minimize sudden weight gain due to water retention, phase out of the diet gradually rather than stop it abruptly: add about 100 to 200 calories to your daily intake and maintain that level for a week or two before adding any more.

To Sum Up

You can lose weight simply by increasing your energy expenditure while holding caloric intake constant, and if you want to keep the weight off, this may be the best approach. Once you reach your goal weight, which may take several months or years of gradually increasing energy expenditure, you will need to increase your caloric intake to maintain that weight. You'll be achieving energy balance on a high-energy throughput, the key to permanent weight control.

If you want to speed up your weight loss, you can follow the dieting recommendations given here or in other books (but avoid radical diets!). The Weight Watchers organization proposes sensible, balanced diets for weight loss. But don't confuse weight *loss* with permanent weight *control.* Most books and organizations emphasize weight *loss.* A low-energy throughput is unlikely to lead to permanent weight control.

Complex carbohydrates and naturally occurring sugars should be the mainstay of your diet. That means plenty of fruits, vegetables and grains, and fewer fatty meats, rich foods, cakes and so on. Carbohydrates are the main energy source during exercise, so your evolving high-energy lifestyle needs plenty of this energy carrier. Eat a variety of foods to make sure that you obtain all the vitamins, minerals and trace elements needed for optimal health.

Most important, enjoy your food. Rather than thinking of food as a kind of enemy, as is common among people with weight problems, think of it as a source of pleasure. By making intelligent food choices so that you derive the maximum pleasure from the calories you take in, and by living a high-energy lifestyle that *requires* you to eat substantial amounts, you'll find mealtimes to be among the highlights of the day—and you won't feel guilty about it.

10

Considerations for Different Groups

The high-energy lifestyle is for everyone—young, old, men, women, the obese, diabetics, even people who have had heart attacks. This chapter outlines some special considerations for each of these groups.

Men, Women and Exercise

There are *some* physical differences between men and women that affect exercise performance and weight loss, although the variability *within* each sex is actually greater than the variability *between* the sexes. So whatever general differences exist between *average* values for males and females don't tell us much about any given individual.

Some differences are caused by sex-linked physiological characteristics, while others are probably the result of differing activity patterns in early life. We can't do much about the biological differences, but we *can* change those that stem from upbringing. For example, it has become much more common than it used to be for women of all ages to take part in sports, and as a result, we can look for some blurring of the difference between the sports performance of the two sexes. In fact, it's already happening: for males, the records are changing by tenths of a second; for females, they're changing by minutes. Probably the most startling figures are the marathon running records. For men, the record has been about 2 hours, 9 minutes for a number of years now, whereas for women it has gone from almost 3 hours down to about 2 hours 25 minutes in the past three or four years. At this rate, women may be doing better than men in another few years! But present knowledge suggests that the very best man is likely to beat the very best woman in most sports.

Before puberty, boys and girls can usually take part in sports on a fairly equal basis. At puberty, changes take place in body structure: men become broader in the shoulders, women in the hips. Men tend to become larger and heavier than women. Women develop more body fat beneath the skin; men have an increase in muscle tissue.

Due to their larger size and greater muscle mass, especially in the upper part of the body, men tend to do much better in power sports such as baseball, football, basketball, racquetball, sprinting, handball —any sports requiring short bursts of energy, leaping or quick changes of direction. But when men and women are subjected to similar programs for improving power, women improve as much as men. In general, though, women do not increase their muscle size as much as men do, possibly because of men's higher concentrations of testosterone, the male sex hormone, which aids in formation of muscle tissue. Of course some women will increase their muscle size much more than others, especially if they train intensively over many years.

Some women worry about increasing their muscle size, thinking it will make them less feminine. But standards of feminity may be changing. The new ideal of feminine beauty, according to a recent *Time* cover story, is "taut, toned and coming on strong." A woman with well-defined muscles and little fat is considered extremely attractive today.

Another important difference between the sexes lies in the amount of body fat they carry, with 25 percent fat being typical among college women, 15 percent fat among college men. Some of this difference is due to natural requirements for maleness and femaleness, but some no doubt results from women's greater tendency to inactivity as a result of early social conditioning. People who live a high-energy lifestyle tend to be less fat regardless of their sex.

Women have a lower resting metabolic rate than men because of their lower amount of lean body mass. A man and woman who weigh the same may find that the woman gains weight on exactly the same diet that allows the man to maintain his weight. So women have an even greater need than men for a high-energy lifestyle if they hope to keep up with men in eating!

Several physiological factors account for sex differences in aerobic endurance. First, men have about 15 percent greater hemoglobin concentration and somewhat higher blood volume and heart volume per unit of body weight than do women. As a result, men have a greater capacity to carry oxygen in the blood, transport it to the various tissues of the body and take away waste products. In addition, women's increased layer of fat beneath the skin interferes somewhat with the ability to liberate heat, which is an important component of endurance exercise. It's more difficult, as a rule, for women to engage in aerobic fitness events. They tend to have a higher heart rate at any given percentage of maximal oxygen consumption, because of their smaller heart size. They also generally have a higher level of perceived exertion.

Since all of these physiological factors change with training, once our society fully accepts the importance of exercise for everyone, we will see relatively small differences between the sexes in sports performance.

Special Considerations for Women

Questions are often raised about the gynecological aspects of exercise for women, the most obvious being whether women should curtail their activity during their menstrual periods. Some women feel uncomfortable during this time and find that engaging in strenuous activity increases their discomfort. In some cases, however, the discomfort is alleviated by exercise. Listen to your body, and you'll soon find out whether you should exercise during your period or not.

During the premenstrual period there is an increase in fluid retention, and some women feel bloated and heavy. This need not prevent you from exercising, though some degree of moderation may be called for.

Some people think strenuous exercise can injure a woman's reproductive organs. If a woman already has a prolapsed uterus or other type of rupture, the organs may slip into the ruptured position during exercise, but the rupture is not *caused* by exercise. A woman whose reproductive structures are normal won't injure them by strenuous activity. In women, ruptures most frequently occur when organs and support structures are overstretched during childbirth, but the second most frequent cause is overweight—another reason to slim down through a high-energy lifestyle.

What about the effect of exercise on the breasts? The ligaments that support the breasts are easily stretched, so wear a good support bra during any kind of active exercise that involves up-and-down movement.

Dr. Rose Frisch of Harvard University has conducted a number of studies that have shown that women who become extremely thin due to intensive physical activity—especially in combination with intensive dieting, as is often the case with ballet dancers and models—may experience cessation of menstrual periods or irregular periods. She has suggested that this may be due to a reduction in body fat below 13 percent or so, the level required for optimal functioning of many systems, including the reproductive system. The body is apparently adjusting to the reduced level of fat by reducing the possibility of conception.

Relatively little is known about the subject, and the menstrual irregularities may be due more to the stress of training or dancing than to the reduction in body fat.

Pregnancy and exercise

Pregnancy is commonly a precursor of obesity, but the reasons aren't entirely clear. Perhaps the habit of eating for two and the decreased physical activity common to many women during pregnancy are carried on after giving birth, partly because the new mother tends to have limited opportunities for exercise.

Moreover, previously thin women tend to become progressively fatter with each cycle of pregnancy and childbirth. During pregnancy the woman stores extra fat in order to be able to sustain the period of lactation. Women who breast-feed their infants return to their pre-pregnancy weight more quickly than those who don't nurse, so our societal tendency not to nurse may be contributing to our increased levels of obesity. This physiological propensity poses a special problem for working mothers who return to work soon after giving birth. They may need to pay extra attention to exercise in order to burn off this extra fat.

There is evidence that women who exercise regularly during pregnancy feel better and have easier deliveries than inactive women. Twenty-four women who ran throughout their pregnancies reported, in a survey done by Judy M. Lutter and Susan Cushman of the University of Minnesota, that running had improved their physical and mental condition. They believed, too, that it shortened their labor and made the pain more tolerable. Strength and flexibility of the trunk muscles, along with the ability to relax, are especially important for delivery.

Exercise for pregnant women may benefit the fetus, too. Offspring of hare and rat mothers that exercised daily during pregnancy were born with larger hearts and better coronary circulation than those born to sedentary mothers. Because of changes in the blood of the mother, the fetus gets more stimulation, which may change the programming of early life, possibly even predisposing the child to activity.

Of course, a pregnant woman shouldn't engage in sports in which the chances of losing balance and falling are very great. But most aerobic activities are not of this type, and there's no evidence that aerobic activity is harmful during pregnancy. In fact, a high-energy throughout is especially important during pregnancy to assure that plenty of necessary nutrients are eaten without excessive weight gain.

The pregnant woman must keep in mind that the extra weight she gains will hamper her performance, and she should expect to slow down a bit as the months go by. But because of the complexity of pregnancy, all questions of exercise should be discussed with the obstetrician, along with other aspects of lifestyle.

The Extremely Obese

A low-energy lifestyle is probably both a cause and an effect of obesity. Moving a very large body is taxing to the circulo-respiratory and musculoskeletal systems, so you avoid moving as much as possible and get into even worse shape. On the other hand, small efforts can lead to large relative improvements. As weight is lost and fitness improves, your working capacity increases faster and faster.

Because the obese have a higher incidence of many diseases, it's important to have medical supervision when starting an exercise program. Keep in mind, too, that severe stress on a deconditioned and unhealthy body can cause serious problems, including, in rare cases, heart attack and sudden death. Of course, *properly undertaken* exercises greatly enhance health. In fact, exercise can normalize many of the hormonal, lipid and blood pressure abnormalities associated with obesity, even if the people don't lose weight.

Obese people have a number of special problems in exercise. They show an increased tendency to exhibit abnormal cardiac function during exercise, due probably to two main factors: a) the enlarged abdomen may force the heart into an unfavorable position; b) the increased blood pressure common in obesity increases the strain on the heart.

The enlarged abdomen can also interfere with the action of the diaphragm and chest wall, leading to breathing difficulties in exercise. The result is extreme breathlessness even in moderate exercise.

Finally, excess fat serves as an insulator, and obese people have a lower density of sweat glands than lean people. The excess weight requires rather large energy release to move the body. As a result, large amounts of heat can build up in the body.

Due to these potential problems, there are several recommendations I would make regarding exercise for the very obese:

1. Swimming is a good initial activity, since it places little strain on joints. The water is a good conductor of heat (providing it isn't too warm), preventing excessive rise in body temperature. If you cannot swim well, there are classes offered by Ys and other organizations.

You can also take exercise classes in the water, thereby putting less strain on your legs. Once the legs and cardiorespiratory system become conditioned in this way, you may be able to exercise more effectively out of water.

2. Stationary cycling is a weight-supported exercise that effectively increases fitness and places relatively little strain on the legs. Many consider it boring, but you can read, watch TV, or talk while you do it. Some cycles allow you to work with both arms and legs at the same time—an especially good way to use calories while enhancing aerobic fitness.

3. Walking puts some strain on the legs, but is well tolerated by almost all obese people. As you become more fit, you must walk faster or up and down hills to get a training effect. Simultaneous vigorous use of the arms in swimming motions adds to the caloric cost of the exercise.

4. Jogging should be undertaken only after several weeks of fast walking without joint pain. Even then, just intersperse a few steps of jogging into each block of walking. If your legs and back respond favorably, then gradually increase the proportion of time spent jogging.

5. In general, keep the exercise intensity just below the anaerobic threshold—be sure you can easily pass the talk test. This will avoid overlarge demands on your heart and lungs. Also, do interval work rather than trying to maintain a continuous strenuous pace. By alternating higher-intensity work of fifteen to sixty seconds duration with similar periods of rest or low-level exercise, you'll be able to do a lot of exercise without placing excessive demands on the aerobic or anaerobic systems.

6. Exercise in cool and well-ventilated areas to assure adequate heat exchange. Remember that exercising in the cold leads to more *fat* loss than exercise in warmer temperatures. Don't overdress on cool days. The sweat must be able to evaporate in order for it to keep you cool. Remove excess clothing as soon as you're warmed up and replace it when you stop. Just tie the extra sweatshirt or jacket around your waist until you need it again.

7. Avoid active competitive sports till your legs are back in shape and your weight is down to a reasonable level. The competition may

lead you to push too hard. Sports requiring jumping and quick changes of direction place a tremendous strain on joints and muscles. Furthermore, if you have gained a lot of weight, your sense of balance may be off, leading you to fall and be injured.

Exercise for People with Handicaps

People with physical or psychological handicaps tend to be extremely inactive, primarily because so much time is devoted to dealing with the handicap that very little is left over for living a high-energy lifestyle. Handicapped people are often obese, too, and subject to the degenerative diseases associated with obesity. For this reason, it's especially important for these people to increase their energy level.

Many people in wheelchairs have in recent years become aware of the importance of physical activity, even to the extent of taking part in long-distance events, including marathons. A number of health clubs and gymnasiums have exercise equipment that can be used with the arms or with one leg. Some of this equipment can be used for activities that promote cardiovascular fitness, such as arm cycling. Swimming or exercise in the water can be beneficial for people who can't easily move themselves around on land.

In the past, exercise was usually associated with sports, and handicapped people find it hard to participate in many sports. But as we become aware that healthful exercise can be noncompetitive and self-paced, it becomes easier for handicapped people to take part in many of the same activities engaged in by the rest of the population.

Exercise for Children

The dominance of cars and television in our society has encouraged our children to be quite inactive. Recent studies of elementary school children's activity throughout the day revealed total energy expenditures to be even lower than was previously thought, especially for girls. One study which measured the heart rate of children throughout the day (by recording it with a portable tape recorder) found that the cardiovascular system was not being stimulated enough to maintain cardiovascular fitness.

All children need a minimum of one hour a day of vigorous aerobic exercise on weekdays and three hours daily on weekends and during vacations. As it is now, our physical education programs favor team sports and competition, which are dominated by the better-skilled and more fit children. As the years progress, the process accelerates and the child with the propensity to obesity becomes even less active and more fat.

Is early activity likely to reduce obesity later in life? Animal studies are very suggestive. When rats exercise during their early life, they gain weight more slowly and level off at a lower weight than rats that live more like the typical American (a comfortable existence with little exercise necessary, and plenty of rat chow to eat). Moreover, the reduced fat stores of the exercised rats are associated with both fewer and smaller fat cells.

Studies on the relation of childhood obesity to adult obesity have not shown a consistent connection. Most obese adults were not obese children, but fat children usually become fat adults.

So the best solution to the problem of childhood obesity, and by extension, adult obesity, is prevention. All children should engage in high-energy lifestyles from the start. The animal studies suggest that this is much more effective than trying to turn the process around later.

School physical education classes and recreational sports groups should focus primarily on aerobic fitness as the foundation for dynamic health. Sports instruction and performance should be aimed at providing skills and attitudes that facilitate a high-energy lifestyle, rather than being viewed as ends in themselves. Whereas we currently spend large amounts of time, money, and experience on the few who are especially talented, all children should be given equal opportunity and encouragement to participate in sports.

Exercise for People Over Sixty

If you've gotten to be past sixty while living a low-energy lifestyle, you've probably put on quite a bit of excess fat, and the health problems associated with inactivity have had a long time to progress, so your level of deconditioning may be extreme. The good news about being in terrible condition (yes, there is some!) is that it's easy to make great progress once you start gently and progress carefully. The health limitations and excess fat are likely to slow you down quite a bit compared with a younger person (though once again, there's a lot of individual variation within this age group). But you may have more leisure time and fewer responsibilities than younger people, and not have to worry about fitting an optimal workout into a limited schedule.

Few older people are inclined to take part in extremely energetic sports. Most take up relatively placid activities like walking, hiking, calisthenics and the less vigorous dance forms. This is sensible in light of the health limitations that have probably resulted from many years of inactivity. In addition, the bones of older people tend to become brittle, though some of this can be reversed by exercise. Consequently, what might be a simple fall in a younger person can result in a life-threatening broken hip in an older person. Fortunately, the quieter activities that older people usually choose are precisely those that I recommend for using up calories and improving aerobic fitness. Even people in their seventies and eighties who start exercise programs are capable of most of the same training effects as are found in younger folks. (For the physiological effects of aging on the human body, see pages 102–105.)

As you progress beyond slow walking and easy swimming, you may want to join a class or center especially aimed at older people. The camaraderie can be pleasant, and you find that others in the class, as well as the instructor, can provide guidelines for you. There are usually a few in every class who have progressed to remarkably high levels, and they can be quite inspirational.

It is wonderful to encounter hardy older people at road races, swimming pools, cross-country ski trails or hiking areas who are enthusiastically living high-energy lives. The evidence isn't yet entirely conclusive, but there is reason to believe they may add some years to their lives in this way. They are definitely adding plenty of life to their years.

Incidentally, the wrinkles that accompany aging are also related to diminished exercise. Studies in Finland and the United States have shown that aerobic exercise makes the skin thicker and stronger, leading to less sagging, wrinkling, and bags under the eyes. These effects are probably due to the increased sweating and blood circulation to the skin which take place during exercise, which in turn increase the nutrients and oxygen available to the skin cells and facilitate removal of waste products. The exercise-induced increase in skin temperature is also important, since the metabolic processes responsible for maintaining healthy skin tissue are enhanced by higher temperatures.

Regular exercise may even improve your sex life. Dr. James White of the University of California at San Diego surveyed 197 middle-aged men about their sexual activity before and after a nine-month aerobic exercise program of an hour a day, four days per week. After the exercise program, the men reported more sexual desire, arousal and orgasms than before. Sexual intercourse, for example, increased from an average of 2.3 times a week before the program to 3.1 times a week at the end of the program.

Dr. White was unsure why these increases took place. Enhanced appearance and self-esteem probably played a role, along with the concrete physiological and hormonal changes associated with improved aerobic fitness.

Exercise for Damaged Hearts

While the value of regular exercise for cardiovascular health is clear (see pages 92–100), the importance of *proper* exercise for many people who already have documented heart disease is even clearer. But note the emphasis on the word *proper*. As we have seen, exercise can be a potent stressor, and someone with an unhealthy heart must be cautious about demanding too much of such a damaged organ.

Putting the issue in bold relief might help. Let's say a person suffers a severe heart attack which brings him close to death. Certainly no one would suggest that he go out for a five-mile run on the following day. On the contrary, as little stress as possible should be imposed in order to allow the repair processes to go forward efficiently, and bed rest is indicated. However, in recent years medical scientists have come to understand that extended bed rest leads to deterioration of many organs and physiological regulatory systems. As a result, some of the most scientifically advanced cardiology and rehabilitation departments routinely put patients who have suffered a myocardial infarction through a progressive series of mild exercises, both in and out of bed. And some put these patients on a treadmill for an exercise tolerance test before they leave the hospital, which might be as little as two weeks after a mild attack. Recently, a leading cardiologist researcher told me how much resistance his unit was encountering from some physicians in implementing the exercise tolerance testing in his hospital, even though the scientific support for the procedure is very convincing. "You have to understand," he said, "that when I did my cardiology training, it was common to put a myocardial infarction patient flat on his back for six weeks after the attack, and many practicing physicians are not aware of how completely attitudes have changed among those in the forefront of knowledge in this area."

The exercise tolerance testing done with these patients does not include strenuous exercise. Rather, the intent is to study the response of the patient to the mild type of exercise he might do when he goes home, such as simply walking around his house or walking stairs. Information derived from this test can help the physician to formulate a more effective therapeutic regimen for the patient.

After leaving the hospital, the patient may be tempted to become what has been called a cardiac cripple, afraid to do almost anything involving exercise, including sexual activity. If the patient does eliminate almost all exertion from his life, there will be continued organic deterioration, and his capacity to do any work will diminish even though the specific damage to his heart may have healed.

The alternative approach is to return to an active life in order to improve dynamic health, and many physicians and cardiac patients are now aware that this is the more sensible approach.

For one thing, the fact that you have a damaged heart is a depressing bit of information, and if you dwell on it, you are likely to be depressed much of the time. On the other hand, if you resolve to improve your total dynamic health in ways that have been shown to work with many other people, your outlook on life is likely to be more optimistic.

Second, the principles of optimal stress described on page 83 also apply to cardiac patients. The optimal stress level is that which stimulates the body to enhance its capacities without being so high as to overwhelm the body's adaptive capacities. Certainly the optimal stress level for a heart patient is likely to be lower than for a person with a healthy heart. But as the heart heals after the infarction, this level increases. Many men who have had myocardial infarctions are now competing regularly in marathons, and the stress imposed by such an event is enormous by any standard. So the level of stress appropriate for cardiac patients is higher than many might suppose. Ironically, a myocardial infarction often serves as a critical incident, alerting the person who has had one to the importance of changing his lifestyle. So he gives up smoking, alters his diet, and exercises regularly, with the result that he becomes healthier than he was before the infarction.

Third, all of the benefits of regular exercise for cardiovascular health mentioned in Chapter 7 are gained by the cardiac patient who exercises. The oxygen supply to the heart improves, the oxygen required by the heart diminishes and the pumping capacity of the heart muscle is enhanced. So postmyocardial infarction patients who are engaged in regular exercise probably have a reduced risk of another infarction and a reduced risk of death compared to similar patients who do not exercise.

Diabetics and Exercise

Diabetes afflicts some ten million Americans, about 5 percent of the population, and its incidence seems to be increasing each year. Diabetes is like other degenerative diseases common in our society in that the disease is already well developed before people even know they have it.

Although diabetes is not fully curable at present, it usually can be controlled fairly well with appropriate diet, medication and exercise. Since these three therapeutic approaches interact with one another, a change in one needs to be coordinated with the others. Therefore, a known diabetic planning to alter his exercise or diet habits should do so in cooperation with his physician, just in case his medication needs adjustment. Even more important, he should become especially well-informed concerning the ways in which exercise and diet influence the different types of diabetes. In this way prevention and control of this disease are primarily where they belong, in the hands of the individual himself.

The diabetic is by no means an invalid who needs to take it easy and avoid any exertion. In fact, he probably has a greater need for exercise as part of his therapeutic regimen than the nondiabetic.

Diabetes is characterized by high levels of blood sugar, or hyperglycemia, to the point where it may spill over into the urine. The disease also involves high levels of blood lipids, so diabetics have an elevated risk of developing coronary heart disease. Diabetes also leads to deterioration of small blood vessels, with gangrene, kidney disorders and blindness as long-term complications.

Medical science distinguishes between juvenile-onset and adult-onset types. Juvenile-onset diabetes is characterized by a deficiency in the production of insulin by the beta cells of the pancreas. One important function of insulin is to facilitate the transport of blood glucose into the muscle cells, where it can be used or stored for later use. If insulin is inadequate, the glucose piles up in the blood to levels several times normal. The individual then uses fats almost exclusively as an energy source, leading to the formation of ketone bodies as metabolic end products. High concentration of ketone bodies make the blood acidic and may lead to diabetic coma.

Juvenile-onset diabetics must usually take insulin injections on a regular basis to bring their blood sugar levels under control. But since the condition is frequently unstable, they must also make sure that their blood sugar levels do not go too low, or they may go into insulin shock. Glucose is the almost exclusive fuel for brain metabolism, and low blood sugar (hypoglycemia) can lead to nausea, dizziness and fainting. In fact, insulin reactions are the most common immediate problem the diabetic must watch for, since they may come on quite rapidly. For this reason, insulin-dependent diabetics frequently carry or keep handy such foods as orange juice and candy to help boost their blood sugar when they feel hypoglycemic.

Exercise can play an important role in the life of a juvenile-onset diabetic, because it has an insulin-like effect on blood sugar, enhancing the uptake of glucose into the muscle cell. In fact, it is important for diabetics to reduce the amount of insulin they take when they exercise, lest they become hypoglycemic.

Adult-onset diabetes is usually identified in later life and comes on gradually. Instead of the insulin levels being low, they are frequently elevated, but the sensitivity of the target organs (the various organs of the body where insulin is used—for example, the muscles) to insulin is decreased. Adult-onset diabetics are almost always overweight, and a program of diet and exercise can often control the problem adequately. Sometimes, orally administered drugs are prescribed to stimulate the secretion of additional insulin by the pancreas. (These drugs are not effective for the juvenile-onset type, since in that condition the beta cells are not functioning properly.) However, recent evidence suggests that such drugs only contribute to a vicious cycle in which the abnormally high insulin levels lead to a further decrease in sensitivity of the target organs, thereby requiring even higher insulin levels. Eventually, the insulin-secreting cells may give out altogether, and the person may become dependent on insulin injections. Therefore, it seems better to limit or eliminate medication for this type of diabetic.

Regular exercise can ameliorate the problems of adult-onset diabetes in four ways. First, it increases the sensitivity of the target organs to insulin; active people tend to have a reduced insulin response to a glucose challenge. Second, it helps glucose enter the muscle cells, thereby lowering its level in the blood. Third, exercise can help control body weight, which is often the cause of the hyperglycemia. And fourth, exercise has a favorable effect on cholesterol and triglycerides, which are often problems in adult diabetes.

Exercise and People with Lung Disease

The two main categories of lung disease that we need to consider are chronic obstructive lung disease (COLD) and asthma. Emphysema and chronic bronchitis fall within the COLD category, and since they're frequently both present in a pulmonary patient, it's convenient to discuss them together. In a healthy lung, each alveolus (small air sac) is surrounded by capillaries, thereby allowing easy diffusion of oxygen into the blood and carbon dioxide into the air. When a person has emphysema, the walls of the alveoli break down and the air sacs become larger but fewer in number. The surface area available for gas exchange diminishes and the exchange of gases is incomplete.

Bronchitis is an inflammation of the bronchi and bronchioles, which results in the accumulation of large amounts of the fluid that lines these airways. In addition, the smooth muscle in the lining of the airways becomes irritated and may contract spasmodically.

Chronic bronchitis is a degenerative disease frequently found in older people along with emphysema. The causes of these diseases are not completely understood, but exposure to air pollution and smoking for many years seems to play an important role. A rather discouraging aspect of these diseases is that they appear to be irreversible.

Strenuous exercise can make us breathless even when our lungs are healthy. The COLD patient may find it impossible to walk more than a block or two before suffering uncomfortable breathlessness, and for this reason, most COLD patients limit their exercise severely. Unfortunately, this makes the situation worse by allowing the deterioration of the many systems of the body that need some stimulation in order to function properly.

The COLD patient must find ways to exercise that will not result in an excessive or uncomfortable need to breathe. The two key words are *aerobic* and *intermittent.* Exercise intense enough so that the aerobic pathways cannot liberate all the necessary energy will require some anaerobic energy release. The lactic acid formed leads to a powerful drive to breathe that may be extremely uncomfortable for a COLD patient. But if the intensity of the exercise is kept low, all of the necessary energy can be liberated aerobically, and the respiratory system will be stimulated only modestly. Alternatively, intermittent bouts of exercise lasting ten to fifteen seconds followed by rest intervals of a similar length can be continued for relatively long periods of time without excessive breathlessness.

Another strategy used with COLD patients is to have them exercise while breathing air with oxygen concentrations of 40 to 60 percent. (Normal air contains about 21 percent oxygen.) Breathing high concentrations of oxygen into the lung allows a given amount of oxygen to be diffused into the blood from a smaller total volume of air. Therefore, the patient finds it possible to exercise at higher intensities before becoming breathless.

Even though the obstructive disease itself is irreversible, the outlook for COLD patients is not altogether bleak. The kind of regular exercise described can have very good effects on the work tolerance and subjective feelings of well-being of these patients. Improved strength and oxidative capacity in the skeletal muscles will result in the ability to do a given amount of work with less strain to the pulmonary and cardiovascular systems. Thus the COLD patient who undertakes a regular exercise program is able to perform normal everyday tasks, including the exercise implicit in them, with less feeling of strain and pulmonary discomfort. While the lungs may not have become healthier, the patient as a whole certainly has.

Unlike COLD, asthma frequently occurs in children and sometimes diminishes in severity or disappears as the person matures. Asthma is characterized by intermittent attacks in which the bronchioles are constricted. Exactly what brings on these attacks is not known.

Although the underlying physiology is unclear, stressful situations often bring on attacks, so one way that regular exercise can help an asthmatic is to reduce the intensity of his normal stress response to the various stressors of life.

But as with COLD, certain types of exercise are beneficial, while other types may be distressing or even life-threatening to an asthmatic. In fact, exercise is sometimes used to provoke an attack as a way of evaluating the severity of the illness. The bronchospasm usually occurs shortly after the cessation of the exercise. The sporadic nature of asthmatic attacks means the physician will seldom be around to observe one unless he provokes it in some way. And doing it systematically under controlled conditions in the office or hospital allows a careful evaluation of various therapeutic techniques.

Dr. Simon Godfrey has done a great deal of excellent research on exercise-induced asthma. In general, he found that the exercise most likely to cause an attack was running, followed by cycling, walking and swimming, in that order. While short bursts of activity can often be tolerated by asthmatic children, continuous running of six to fifteen minutes is very potent in bringing on an attack. Therefore, the continuous aerobic exercise advocated for most people may not be ideal for the asthmatic. Many asthmatics find, however, that they can exercise and still avoid attacks by continuing the aerobic activity for at least 30 minutes, thereby greatly reducing the severity or eliminating the postexercise wheezing: in some way running through it. Since swimming is the least likely of all aerobic activities to provoke an attack, it is the activity of choice. Researchers at Yale University School of Medicine have found that 500 milligrams of vitamin C, taken one and a half hours or less before exercise, tended to reduce exercise-induced asthma attacks.

If a young asthmatic allows himself to become an invalid due to his disability, his well-being for the rest of his life will suffer far more than is warranted by the disease alone: his heart will become weak, his muscles flabby, and so on. But if he finds the right type and intensity of exercise for him, the loss to his total health due to the disease will be small. Thus almost everyone can profit from high-energy living, especially those whose handicaps, age or illness may incline them to sedentary lives, which in turn serve to weaken them further.

Changing Society

Although taking personal responsibility for your own weight and health has been emphasized throughout this book, our social institutions can do a great deal to either limit or facilitate our pursuit of a healthful way of life. Money spent on health-promoting and disease-preventing activities is likely to have a greater impact on our collective health than money spent on more medical technology, drugs and curative medical care.

Many large companies and government agencies have already done something to improve their employees' health by building gymnasiums, swimming pools and running tracks, and staffing them with people trained in exercise physiology, nutrition and stress management. Studies of the people who use these facilities have shown remarkable improvements in health, and the changes have been good for business, too. A study of 1,300 employees at the Prudential Insurance Company of Houston found that exercisers lost an average of 3.5 days per year to illness, compared to 8.6 days for the nonexercisers. Those who exercised also had lower medical bills and were more productive at work. Dr. Donald W. Bowne, the vice-president for medical services, has pointed out that the expenditures for major medical health care are directly related to aerobic fitness. For a recent year studied, those low in fitness generated an average expense of $500, those in the fair level of fitness $580, those at the good level $80, and those at the high level $0 of major medical expense. A five-year exercise program for eight hundred New York state employees improved aerobic fitness, reduced cardiovascular risk factors, and cut employee sick leave by 37 percent. Studies done in the U.S.S.R. have shown that people who exercise regularly are more productive, visit the doctor less often, and are less prone to industrial accidents.

Employees are often permitted to exercise during company time in the hope that increased productivity during the rest of the day will more than compensate for the lost worktime. Employees may take shorter lunch hours and breaks to make up the time, or exercise before or after work.

But most employed people don't work in companies or agencies that have their own exercise facilities. How can employers promote high-energy lifestyles for them? Here are some of the things they can do:

* Share the cost for enrollment at Ys, health clubs, and other such facilities.
* Collaborate with other businesses in supporting private or public exercise facilities.
* Make time available (flex-time) for exercise.
* Provide shower facilities so people can walk/run/cycle to or from work.
* Consider lifestyle when hiring and promoting, given its implications for productivity, longevity, health-care costs and replacement costs. For example, it's extremely expensive to replace an executive who is stricken with coronary heart disease at age fifty, just when his value to the company is at its peak.

What Else Can Society Do?

Unions can negotiate high-energy-lifestyle features into contracts.

Life insurance and health insurance companies such as Blue Cross can adjust their premiums to take account of exercise and obesity. They already do this for smoking, and some are beginning to give discounts to regular exercisers.

Food companies can reduce sugar, fat and salt in processed foods, as some are starting to do.

The government can foster research and education of the public on exercise and nutrition, and can provide scholarships and loans for students training for careers in exercise physiology and nutrition.

The media can help by building health concepts into regular programming, and by doing educational specials, perhaps in connection with sports events, to encourage participation along with spectatorship. Less advertising of foods high in fat, sugar and salt could have an impact.

School systems can make children aware of the importance of establishing a high-energy lifestyle early in life, for lifelong health. They can emphasize aerobics in physical education programs, teach concepts of exercise, nutrition and weight control, and improve nutrition in school lunches. They can keep school gyms and pools open and staffed in the afternoons and evenings; these are community resources that are usually locked up during the hours when many children and adults could use them. Schools can offer adult education courses in weight control, exercise and nutrition, perhaps in collaboration with local medical societies and recreation agencies. And they can include material on exercise throughout the curriculum, in biology, health and physical education courses, from elementary school through college. Teachers should have continuing education in exercise physiology and nutrition.

Senior citizens' residences and groups should emphasize exercise.

Religious groups can foster a high-energy lifestyle through church activities.

Recreation departments and parks agencies should provide attractive running, swimming, walking and cycling areas, publicize them, and hold special events.

Medical systems and agencies such as the American Heart Association and the American Cancer Society can contribute as well. I am a member of the Exercise Committee of the New York Heart Association, and under the leadership of Dr. Lenore Zohman we have engaged in several health promotion activities. For example, we made up and distributed exercise maps of the five boroughs of New York City, so that New Yorkers and visitors will know where they can go to do aerobic exercise. We also wrote a booklet providing guidelines for people selecting facilities for exercise stress testing and aerobic exercise.

Medical schools should increase their coverage of exercise in their courses, perhaps by seeking funds for special faculty positions, as has been done for other areas such as nutrition and geriatrics.

The main role of physicians will continue to be care of people with manifest disease, since many health promotion/disease prevention activities are largely educational in nature and can be effectively carried out by health educators, nurses, exercise physiologists, nutritionists and psychologists. But physicians occupy a special place in our society, and many people report that the main reason they decided to change their health behavior was that their physicians told them to. In a sense that is the official word, since the physician is not trying to sell the patient any one idea, as people who write books pushing a particular kind of exercise, a new diet, or megadoses of vitamins often are.

Even though it is probably not cost-effective for doctors to spend a lot of time educating individual patients about exercise and nutrition, they can support the importance of high-energy living and refer patients to appropriate professionals when necessary. In group practices, it might be possible to employ a health professional for the task of education. Perhaps with some additional training nurses could play this role.

Our best hope for the future is to develop in young children the attitudes, knowledge and physical ability needed to maintain a high-energy lifestyle for the rest of their lives. Even though you can change your behavior at any age, it is probably better to avoid falling into a low-energy lifestyle in the first place.

If we as a society create the framework which will make a high-energy lifestyle the normal way to live, it will be much easier for individuals to adopt this healthier, saner, more joyful way of life. Very few things would give me more satisfaction than knowing that people were using the concepts in this book to promote not only their own personal health but also the health of their families and communities.

Appendix

Guidelines for Body Weight
(height without shoes and weight without clothes)

HEIGHT *(feet and inches)*	WEIGHT *(pounds)*			
	Men		Women	
	Average	Acceptable	Average	Acceptable
4 10			102	92–119
4 11			104	94–122
5 0			107	96–125
5 1			110	99–128
5 2	123	112–141	113	102–131
5 3	127	115–144	116	105–134
5 4	130	118–148	120	108–138
5 5	133	121–152	123	111–142
5 6	136	124–156	128	114–146
5 7	140	128–161	132	118–150
5 8	145	132–166	136	122–154
5 9	149	136–170	140	126–158
5 10	153	140–174	144	130–163
5 11	158	144–179	148	134–168
6 0	162	148–184	152	138–173
6 1	166	152–189		
6 2	171	156–194		
6 3	176	160–199		
6 4	181	164–204		

SOURCE: G. Bray, ed., *Obesity in America,* NIH publication No. 80-359 (1980).

Percent of U.S. Population
Deviating from Desirable Weight

| Age | MEN | | WOMEN | |
---	10–19 percent	20 percent or more	10–19 percent	20 percent or more
20–74	18.1	14.0	12.6	23.8
20–24	11.1	7.4	9.8	9.6
25–34	16.7	13.6	8.1	17.1
35–44	22.1	17.0	12.3	24.3
45–54	19.9	15.8	15.1	27.8
55–64	18.9	15.1	15.5	34.7
65–74	19.1	13.4	17.5	31.5

SOURCE: G. Bray, ed., *Obesity in America,* NIH publication No. 80-359 (1980).

Approximate Energy Expenditure in Selected
Activities for People of Different Weights
(Calories per minute)

| ACTIVITY | WEIGHT *(pounds)* | | | | | |
---	110	130	150	170	190	210
Aerobic dancing						
"walking pace"	3.3	3.8	4.4	5.0	5.6	6.2
"jogging pace"	5.3	6.2	7.1	8.1	9.0	10.0
"running pace"	6.8	8.0	9.2	10.5	11.7	12.9
Archery	3.3	3.8	4.4	5.0	5.6	6.2
Badminton	4.9	5.7	6.6	7.5	8.3	9.2
Basketball	6.9	8.1	9.4	10.6	11.9	13.2
Billiards	2.1	2.5	2.9	3.2	3.6	4.0
Canoeing—leisure	2.2	2.6	3.0	3.4	3.8	4.2
Canoeing—racing	5.2	6.1	7.0	7.9	8.9	9.8

ACTIVITY	WEIGHT *(pounds)*					
	110	130	150	170	190	210
Carpentry	2.6	3.1	3.5	4.0	4.5	4.9
Carpet sweeping	2.3	2.7	3.2	3.6	4.0	4.5
Circuit training	9.3	10.9	12.6	14.2	15.9	17.6
Croquet	3.0	3.5	4.0	4.5	5.1	5.6
Cycling—5.5 mph	3.2	3.8	4.4	4.9	5.5	6.1
Cycling—9.4 mph	5.0	5.9	6.8	7.7	8.6	9.5
Dancing—ballroom	2.6	3.0	3.5	3.9	4.4	4.8
Dancing—disco	5.2	6.1	7.0	7.9	8.9	9.8
Farming						
barn cleaning	6.8	8.0	9.2	10.4	11.6	12.8
driving tractor	1.9	2.2	2.5	2.8	3.2	3.5
milking by hand	2.7	3.2	3.7	4.2	4.6	5.1
milking by machine	1.2	1.4	1.6	1.8	2.0	2.2
Field hockey	6.7	7.9	9.1	10.3	11.5	12.7
Gardening						
(digging, hedging,						
mowing, raking)	5.0	5.9	6.8	7.7	8.6	9.5
Golf	4.3	5.0	5.8	6.5	7.3	8.1
Horse riding						
galloping	6.9	8.1	9.3	10.6	11.8	13.0
trotting	5.5	6.5	7.5	8.5	9.5	10.5
walking	2.1	2.4	2.8	3.2	3.5	3.9
Judo	9.8	11.5	13.3	15.0	16.8	18.6
Lying or						
sitting down	1.1	1.3	1.5	1.7	1.9	2.1
Mopping floor	3.2	3.5	4.0	4.6	5.1	5.7
Music playing						
accordion (sitting)	1.6	1.9	2.2	2.5	2.8	3.0
conducting	2.0	2.3	2.7	3.0	3.4	3.7
drums (sitting)	3.3	3.9	4.5	5.1	5.7	6.3
piano (sitting)	2.0	2.4	2.7	3.1	3.4	3.8
violin (sitting)	2.3	2.7	3.1	3.5	3.9	4.3
woodwind (sitting)	1.6	1.9	2.2	2.5	2.8	3.0

ACTIVITY	WEIGHT *(pounds)*					
	110	130	150	170	190	210
Running						
11.5 minutes per mile	6.8	8.0	9.2	10.5	11.7	12.9
9 minutes per mile	9.7	11.4	13.1	14.9	16.6	18.4
7 minutes per mile	12.2	13.9	15.6	17.4	19.1	20.8
5.5 minutes per mile	14.5	17.1	19.7	22.3	24.9	27.6
Skiing, cross-country	7.2	8.4	9.7	11.0	12.3	13.6
Standing quietly	1.3	1.5	1.7	1.9	2.2	2.4
Swimming						
backstroke	8.5	10.0	11.5	13.0	14.5	16.2
breast stroke	8.1	9.6	11.0	12.5	13.9	15.5
crawl	6.4	7.6	8.7	9.9	11.0	12.2
Table tennis	3.4	4.0	4.6	5.2	5.8	6.5
Tennis	5.5	6.4	7.4	8.4	9.4	10.4
Volleyball	2.5	3.0	3.4	3.9	4.3	4.8
Walking						
3 miles per hour	3.4	3.8	4.2	4.6	5.1	5.5
4 miles per hour	4.0	4.7	5.4	6.2	6.9	7.6
Window cleaning	2.9	3.4	3.9	4.5	5.0	5.5

SOURCE: Various publications

Weight Loss per Year *or* Additional Calories You Can Eat per Day,
as a Result of Three Hours a Week of Some Common Activities*
(Amounts for a 150-pound woman [upper line] or 200-pound man [lower line])

Activity	Calories per minute	Weight loss per year (pounds)	Calories per day	Equivalent food
Bicycling				
(5.5 mph)	5.0	13.4	129	1 cupcake
	6.5	17.4	169	3 ounces roast beef
Bowling (nonstop)	6.7	17.9	172	1 hot dog
	9.0	24.1	231	1 cup fruit-flavored yogurt
Golf (foursome)	4.0	10.7	103	1 cup lemonade
	5.5	14.7	141	1 ounce corn chips
Racquetball	9.0	24.1	231	3 ounces broiled lean steak
	11.7	31.1	301	1 piece apple pie
Running (5.5 mph)	10.8	28.9	278	slice lemon meringue pie
	14.2	38	365	2 hamburgers
Skiing (cross-country)	11.7	31.1	301	1 pound grapes
	15.8	42.3	406	½ cup almonds
Swimming (crawl, 20 yards a minute)	4.8	12.8	123	10 potato chips
	6.3	16.8	162	1 ounce chocolate-coated peanuts
Tennis	6.7	17.9	172	2 rolls
	9.2	24.6	237	2 ounces fudge

Activity	Calories per minute	Weight loss per year (pounds)	Calories per day	Equivalent food
Dancing (vigorous)	5.7	15.2	147	1 English muffin
	7.5	20.1	193	½ cup chocolate pudding
Walking (4 mph)	6.2	16.1	159	1 slice pizza
	8.1	21.7	208	¼ cup peanuts
Horseback riding	6.7	17.9	172	2 cups cherries
	9.0	24.1	231	2½ ounces mayonnaise
Farm chores	3.8	10.2	98	1 banana
	5.1	13.6	131	12 ounces cola
Shoveling snow	7.8	20.9	201	1 ounce butter
	10.7	26.7	257	1 cup dried prunes
Washing floors	4.6	12.3	126	½ cup sherbet
	6.0	16.0	154	1 cup milk
Dusting	2.7	7.2	69	1 pancake
	3.5	9.4	86	3½ ounces wine
Cooking	3.9	10.4	100	1 cup buttermilk
	5.2	13.9	134	½ cup strawberry ice cream

Expected Weight Loss from 240 Minutes
of Running per Week at Speed of 7 Miles per Hour

	Height (feet and inches)	Starting Weight	Desirable Weight	Calories used/minute	Pounds lost per week	Weeks needed to lose 10 pounds	Weeks needed to lose 30 pounds	Weeks needed to lose 50 pounds
FEMALES	5 0	117	107	9	.62	16		
		137		11	.75		40	
		157		13	.89			56
	5 3	126	116	10	.69	15		
		146		12	.82		37	
		166		14	.96			52
	5 6	138	128	11	.75	13		
		158		13	.89		34	
		178		15	1.03			49
MALES	5 7	150	140	12	.82	12		
		170		14	.96		31	
		190		16	1.10			45
	5 10	163	153	13	.89	11		
		183		15	1.03		29	
		203		17	1.17			43
	6 1	176	166	14	.96	10		
		196		16	1.10		27	
		216		18	1.23			41

Expected Weight Loss
from 240 Minutes of Aerobic Dancing per Week

Height (feet and inches)	Starting Weight	Desirable Weight	Calories used/minute	Pounds lost per week	Weeks needed to lose 10 pounds	30 pounds	50 pounds
FEMALES							
5 0	117	107	5.6	.38	26		
	137		6.5	.45		67	
	157		7.4	.51			98
5 3	126	116	6.0	.41	24		
	146	1	7.0	.48		63	
	166		7.9	.54			93
5 6	138	128	6.6	.45	22		
	158		7.6	.52		58	
	178		8.5	.58			86
MALES							
5 7	150	140	7.1	.49	20		
	170		8.1	.56		54	
	190		9.0	.62			81
5 10	163	153	7.8	.53	19		
	183		8.7	.60		50	
	203		9.7	.67			75
6 1	176	166	8.4	.58	17		
	196		9.4	.64		47	
	216		10.3	.71			70

Expected Weight Loss from 240 Minutes
of Cycling per Week at Speed of 9.4 mph

	Height (feet and inches)	Starting Weight	Desirable Weight	Calories used/minute	Pounds lost per week	Weeks needed to lose		
						10 pounds	30 pounds	50 pounds
FEMALES	5 0	117	107	5.3	.36	28		
		137		6.2	.42		71	
		157		7.1	.48			104
	5 3	126	116	5.7	.39	26		
		146		6.6	.45		67	
		166		7.5	.51			98
	5 6	138	128	6.2	.43	23		
		158		7.1	.49		61	
		178		8.0	.55			91
MALES	5 7	150	140	6.8	.47	21		
		170		7.7	.53		57	
		190		8.6	.59			85
	5 10	163	153	7.3	.50	20		
		183		8.2	.56		54	
		203		9.1	.62			81
	6 1	176	166	7.9	.54	19		
		196		8.8	.60		50	
		216		9.7	.67			75

Expected Weight Loss from 420 Minutes
of Walking per Week at Speed of 4 mph

	Height (feet and inches)	Starting Weight	Desirable Weight	Calories used/minute	Pounds lost per week	Weeks needed to lose 10 pounds	30 pounds	50 pounds
FEMALES	5 0	117	107	4.2	.51	20		
		137		4.9	.59		51	
		157		5.7	.68			74
	5 3	126	116	4.5	.54	19		
		146		5.3	.63		48	
		166		6.0	.72			69
	5 6	138	128	5.0	.60	17		
		158		5.7	.68		44	
		178		6.4	.77			65
MALES	5 7	150	140	5.4	.65	15		
		170		6.2	.74		41	
		190		6.9	.83			60
	5 10	163	153	5.9	.71	14		
		183		6.6	.79		38	
		203		7.4	.89			56
	6 1	176	166	6.4	.77	13		
		196		7.1	.85		35	
		216		7.8	.94			53

Expected Weight Loss from 240 Minutes
of Swimming per Week at Speed of 36 Yards per Minute

Height (feet and inches)	Starting Weight	Desirable Weight	Calories used/minute	Pounds lost per week	Weeks needed to lose		
					10 pounds	30 pounds	50 pounds
FEMALES							
5 0	117	107	9	.62	16		
	137		10	.69		43	
	157		11	.75			67
5 3	126	116	9	.62	16		
	146		10.5	.72		42	
	166		12	.82			61
5 6	138	128	10	.69	15		
	158		11.5	.79		38	
	178		13	.89			56
MALES							
5 7	150	140	11	.75	13		
	170		12.5	.86		35	
	190		14	.96			52
5 10	163	153	11.5	.79	13		
	183		13	.89		34	
	203		14.5	.99			51
6 1	176	166	12.5	.86	12		
	196		14	.96		31	
	216		15.5	1.06			47

Approximate Weight Loss in a Year
for Ten People on Various Activity Programs*

Sex	Age	Height	Weight	Desirable Weight	Activity	Expected Yearly Loss
F	35	5'4"	140	120	Aerobic dancing, 1 hour, 3 times a week	20
M	30	6'0"	210	162	Circuit training and stationary cycling, 45 minutes, 4 times a week	30
M	60	5'10"	175	153	Walking, 90 minutes a day	53†
F	60	5'2"	125	113	Walking, 90 minutes a day	37†
F	45	5'6"	150	128	Swimming, 45 minutes 3 times a week	20
M	50	5'8"	170	145	Cycling, 240 minutes a week	21
F	25	5'5"	135	123	Running, 40 minutes 4 times a week	26†
M	27	5'9"	180	149	Running, 240 minutes a week	46†
F	40	5'3"	175	116	Walking, 1 hour, 5 times a week	25
F	23	5'8"	145	136	Racquetball, 1 hour, 4 times a week	32†

*Expected yearly loss will vary according to metabolic differences between individuals and caloric intake of each individual. If you are not fit, it may take a few weeks for you to do the activity vigorously, so your weight loss will be slow at first and accelerate as you get more fit and active. Heavier people use more calories to transport their bodies, allowing weight to be lost a bit faster.

†Since this amount of weight loss would be excessive, these people would need to increase their calorie intake appropriately.

How to Estimate Your Percent Body Fat Using Skinfolds

About half your total fat is stored just below the skin, so by measuring the thickness of four selected skinfolds, including the underlying fat, and by locating the sum of the four in the accompanying table, you can arrive at an estimate of the percent of your body weight composed of fat.

You'll need a set of calipers to measure your skinfolds in millimeters, and another person to take the actual measurements. You can purchase calipers for about $10 from Health and Education Services, 2422 Irving Park Road, Chicago, Illinois 60613.

The measurements are made on one side of the body. Grasp the skinfold between the thumb and forefinger; include skin and underlying fat, but not the muscle. Put the calipers where your fingers are. Take two readings at each site, and if they differ by more than .5 millimeters, take at least one more, using the mean of the two closest readings as the value for that site. Between measurements, release and then regrasp the skinfold.

The anatomical landmarks for the skinfold measures are:

Biceps—halfway between armpits and elbow joint.

Triceps—halfway between shoulder and elbow. The biceps and triceps skinfolds are made with arm hanging down in a relaxed position.

Iliac crest—just over the hipbone at the side of the body.

Subscapula—the bottom point of the shoulder blade.

Add the figures for the biceps, triceps, iliac crest and subscapula skinfolds, find that sum in the skinfolds column, and read the estimated percent from the appropriate age and sex column. For example, a female age thirty-five with a skinfold sum of 50 would have a percent fat of about 28.2.

College-age men and women in the United States average 25 and 15 percent fat, respectively. These averages are probably a bit too high from the standpoint of health and appearance; women should have between 15 and 20 percent fat, men between 10 and 15 percent. Since there is no known biological advantage to our tendency to get fatter as we get older, you should maintain your thinness throughout life. Note in the table that the same sum of skinfolds is associated with a greater percent body fat as one ages, because lean tissue is being replaced by fat stored throughout the body, not only beneath the skin. However, this table was not specifically based on highly active people, who tend to retain their lean tissues.

Determination of Percent Body Fat from the Sum of the Biceps, Triceps, Subscapula and Iliac Skinfolds

Skinfolds (mm)	Males (age in years)				Females (age in years)			
	17–29	30–39	40–49	50+	16–29	30–39	40–49	50+
15	4.8	—	—	—	10.5	—	—	—
20	8.1	12.2	12.2	12.6	14.1	17.0	19.8	21.4
25	10.5	14.2	15.0	15.6	16.8	19.4	22.2	24.0
30	12.9	16.2	17.7	18.6	19.5	21.8	24.5	26.6
35	14.7	17.7	19.6	20.8	21.5	23.7	26.4	28.5
40	16.4	19.2	21.4	22.9	23.4	25.5	28.2	30.3
45	17.7	20.4	23.0	24.7	25.0	26.9	29.6	31.9
50	19.0	21.5	24.6	26.5	26.5	28.2	31.0	33.4
55	20.1	22.5	25.9	27.9	27.8	29.4	32.1	34.6
60	21.2	23.5	27.1	29.2	29.1	30.6	33.2	35.7
65	22.2	24.3	28.2	30.4	30.2	31.6	34.1	36.7
70	23.1	25.1	29.3	31.6	31.2	32.5	35.0	37.7
75	24.0	25.9	30.3	32.7	32.2	33.4	35.9	38.7
80	24.8	26.6	31.2	33.8	33.1	34.3	36.7	39.6
85	25.5	27.2	32.1	34.8	34.0	35.1	37.5	40.4
90	26.2	27.8	33.0	35.8	34.8	35.8	38.3	41.2
95	26.9	28.4	33.7	36.6	35.6	36.5	39.0	41.9
100	27.6	29.0	34.4	37.4	36.4	37.2	39.7	42.6
105	28.2	29.6	35.1	38.2	37.1	37.9	40.4	43.3
110	28.8	30.1	35.8	39.0	37.8	38.6	41.0	43.9

Skinfolds	Males (age in years)				Females (age in years)			
(mm)	17–29	30–39	40–49	50+	16–29	30–39	40–49	50+
115	29.4	30.6	36.4	39.7	38.4	39.1	41.5	44.5
120	30.0	31.1	37.0	40.4	39.0	39.6	42.0	45.1
125	30.5	31.5	37.6	41.1	39.6	40.1	42.5	45.7
130	31.0	31.9	38.2	41.8	40.2	40.6	43.0	46.2
135	31.5	32.3	38.7	42.4	40.8	41.1	43.5	46.7
140	32.0	32.7	39.2	43.0	41.3	41.6	44.0	47.2
145	32.5	33.1	39.7	43.6	41.8	42.1	44.5	47.7
150	32.9	33.5	40.2	44.1	42.3	42.6	45.0	48.2
155	33.3	33.9	40.7	44.6	42.8	43.1	45.4	48.7
160	33.7	34.3	41.2	45.1	43.3	43.6	45.8	49.2
165	34.1	34.6	41.6	45.6	43.7	44.0	46.2	49.6
170	34.5	34.8	42.0	46.1	44.1	44.4	46.6	50.0
175	34.9	—	—	—	44.8	47.0	50.4
180	35.3	—	—	—	45.2	47.4	50.8
185	35.6	—	—	—	45.6	47.8	51.2
190	35.9	—	—	—	45.9	48.2	51.6
195	—	—	—	—	46.2	48.5	52.0
200	—	—	—	—	46.5	48.8	52.4
205	—	—	—	—	—	49.1	52.7
210	—	—	—	—	—	49.4	53.0

In two-thirds of the instances the error was within ± 3.5 percent of the body weight as fat for the women and ± 5 percent for the men.

SOURCE: Adapted from "Body Fat Assessed from Total Body Density and Its Estimation from Skinfold Thickness" by J.V.G.A. Durnin and J. Womersley, *British Journal of Nutrition*, Vol. 32 (1974), p. 95.

NUTRITIONAL VALUES OF CERTAIN FAST FOODS*

	Serving size (oz.)	Calories	Fat (gm.)	Carbohydrates (gm.)	Total sugars (gm.)	Sodium (mg.)	Percentage RDA†									
							Protein	Vitamin A	Thiamin	Riboflavin	Vitamin B6	Vitamin B12	Niacin	Calcium	Phosphorus	Iron
HAMBURGERS																
Burger King Whopper	9	660	41	49	9	1083	57%	12%	51%	30%	19%	67%	55%	9%	29%	26%
Jack-in-the-Box Jumbo Jack	8¼	538	28	44	7	1007	61	9	56	41	13	70	57	13	29	24
McDonald's Big Mac	7½	591	33	46	6	963	59	5	52	33	13	63	55	23	44	23
Wendy's Old Fashioned	6½	413	22	29	5	708	52	8	36	26	13	83	45	8	24	27
SANDWICHES																
Roy Rogers Roast Beef Sandwich	5½	356	12	34	0	610	63	5	38	29	16	37	60	2	28	23
Burger King Chopped-Beef Steak Sandwich	6¾	445	13	50	0.7	966	67	5	48	34	25	40	66	15	37	30
Hardee's Roast Beef Sandwich	4½	351	17	32	3	765	41	4	36	22	10	47	42	8	29	17
Arby's Roast Beef Sandwich	5¼	370	15	36	1	869	52	4	36	21	10	53	56	5	35	20

FISH	Long John Silver's	7½	483	27	27	0.1	1333	72	5	17	12	16	133	24	3	46	3
	Arthur Treacher's Original	5¼	439	27	27	0.3	421	46	3	11	6	10	27	18	2	32	3
	McDonald's Filet-o-Fish	4½	383	18	38	3	613	35	3	39	19	6	23	25	14	27	9
	Burger King Whaler	7	584	34	50	5	968	48	3	38	20	7	60	31	8	50	12
CHICKEN	Kentucky Fried Chicken Snack Box	6¾	405	21	16	0	728	78	4	21	25	19	40	72	6	35	14
	Arthur Treacher's Original Chicken	5½	409	23	25	0	580	57	3	12	10	24	10	87	2	33	4
SPECIALTIES	Wendy's Chili	10	266	9	29	9	1190	50	54	20	169	18	47	8	9	27	27
	Pizza Hut Pizza Supreme	7¾‡	506	15	64	6	1281	61	36	59	40	17	43	49	41	46	24
	Jack-in-the-Box Taco	5⅝§	429	26	34	3	926	35	25	16	13	15	27	18	20	33	12

*As analyzed for the September 1979 issue of Consumer Reports. Formulations of these foods may have been changed since that time.
†Recommended Daily Allowance for an adult woman, as set by the National Academy of Sciences/National Research Council.
‡One-half of a 15½-oz. 10-in. Pizza Supreme Thin and Crispy.
§Two 2¾-oz. tacos.

SOURCE: *Consumer Reports*, September 1979. Copyright 1979 by Consumers Union of United States, Inc., Mount Vernon, New York 10550. Reprinted by permission.

Percent of Total Calories
Represented by Protein, Fat and Carbohydrate

Food	Calories	Percent Protein	Percent Fat	Percent Carbo-hydrate
FRUITS				
1 medium apple	90	1	9	90
½ cup apple juice	50	1	—	99
⅔ cup blueberries	60	1	3	96
15 large raw cherries	70	8	3.5	88.5
12 medium dates	275	2.5	1.5	96
½ medium grapefruit	40	4	2	94
6 ounces grapefruit juice	75	4.7	2.3	93
22–24 grapes	70	4.5	12	83.5
½ of 4½-inch cantaloupe	30	8	2.5	89.5
½ cup cubed watermelon	25	7	6.5	86.5
1 medium orange	75	7.5	3.5	90
6 ounces orange juice	80	5	4	91
1 medium peach	45	6	2	92
6 ounces unsweetened pineapple juice	100	2.7	1.7	95.6
2 medium plums	50	3.9	3.5	92.6
¼ cup raisins	115	3.1	.7	96.2
⅔ cup raw strawberries	35	5.5	3.1	91.4
VEGETABLES				
6–7 fresh asparagus stalks	20	31	7	62
½ avocado	170	4.5	71	24.5
½ cup grated raw carrot	20	10	4	86
2 large stalks celery	15	17.5	4.5	78
1 small ear corn	90	13	8.5	78.5
½ medium cucumber	7	12	9	79
½ cup cooked lentils	105	30	—	70
⅕ head iceberg lettuce	12	20	5.6	74.4
3½ ounces raw mushrooms	30	35	9	56
1 tablespoon chopped onion	4	18	—	82

Food	Calories	Percent Protein	Percent Fat	Percent Carbo-hydrate
½ cup cooked drained green peas	55	30	4.5	65.5
1 medium green pepper	15	20	5.5	74.5
1 large pickle	15	19.6	14.8	65.6
1 medium baked potato	95	10.5	1	88.5
20 french-fried potatoes	275	6.5	42	51.5
4 small radishes	7	28.6	—	71.4
½ cup drained spinach	20	45	10.1	44.9
½ cup boiled summer squash	15	21.8	5.5	72.7
1 medium tomato	35	15.1	4.5	80.4
6 ounces tomato juice	35	15.1	4.5	80.4
½ cup fresh lima beans	90	26	4	70
¾ cup fresh or frozen green beans	25	22	6	72
⅔ cup broccoli	25	34.5	8	57.5
BREADS, CEREALS, PASTA, RICE				
1 slice rye bread	55	13	6	81
1 slice white bread	60	13	10	77
1 slice whole wheat bread	55	16.5	10.5	73
¾ cup 40% bran flakes	90	10.7	4	85.3
1 cup corn flakes	95	8.6	1	90.4
1 large shredded wheat biscuit	140	11	.6	88.4
¾ cup oatmeal	65	12	14	74
¾ cup Cream of Wheat	50	16	2	82
2 Ry-Krisp wafers	45	12	4	84
1 4-inch pancake	50	13	19	68
1 cup cooked macaroni or spaghetti	155	13	3.5	83.5
⅔ cup brown rice, cooked	120	8.4	4.5	87.1
⅔ cup white rice, cooked	110	7.6	.9	91.5
1 large hamburger bun	115	11	16	73
1 large hard roll	160	12.4	11.1	76.5
1 4½ × 5½ × ½-inch waffle	205	12.6	35	52.4
1 tablespoon wheat germ	35	25.6	23.1	51.3

Food	Calories	Percent Protein	Percent Fat	Percent Carbo-hydrate
NUTS				
12–15 whole almonds	90	12.5	75	12.5
15–17 shelled roasted peanuts	90	16	72	12
1 tablespoon peanut butter	90	16	72	12
2 tablespoons chopped pecans	105	3.6	89	7.4
OILS, DRESSINGS, SAUCES				
1 tablespoon mayonnaise	100	.8	98	1.2
¼ cup Hollandaise sauce	180	5	94	1
1 tablespoon ketchup	20	6.6	5	88.4
1 tablespoon vegetable oil	125	—	100	—
DAIRY PRODUCTS				
1 ounce Cheddar cheese	120	24.5	73.5	2
¼ cup creamed cottage cheese	60	54	32	14
1 ounce cream cheese	110	9	89	2
1 ounce Swiss cheese	110	31.5	66.5	2
6 ounce cocoa made with milk	174	15	43	42
¼ cup half-and-half	80	9.5	76	14.5
¼ cup heavy cream	210	2.7	93.7	3.6
¼ cup light cream	130	6	84.5	9.5
1 large boiled egg	80	31.7	66	2.3
8 ounces whole milk	160	21	50	29
8 ounces low-fat (2%) milk	150	31	32	37
8 ounces skim milk or buttermilk	90	40	2	58
8 ounces plain yogurt	125	28	30	42
1 tablespoon butter	100	—	100	—
MEAT AND FISH				
3 strips bacon	155	21	78	2
¼ pound broiled hamburger	245	35	65	—
4½ × 2½ × 1-inch sirloin, broiled	410	22	78	—

Food	Calories	Percent Protein	Percent Fat	Percent Carbo- hydrate
½ fried chicken breast	205	68	28	4
1 fried chicken thigh and drumstick	235	51	43.6	5.4
4 ounces steamed flounder or sole	200	62.5	37.5	—
4 ounces fried haddock	165	50	34.6	15.4
3½ ounces broiled salmon	180	63	37	—
⅝ cup tuna in oil (drained)	195	61.7	38.3	—
⅝ cup tuna in water	125	94	6	—
⅔ cup lobster meat	95	79.4	19.3	1.3
3½ ounces smoked ham	290	30	70	—
3½ ounces broiled lamb chop	360	25	75	—
3½ ounces light meat turkey	175	78.6	21.4	—
3½ ounces dark meat turkey	205	62.5	37.5	—
3½ ounces broiled veal cutlet	215	52.2	47.8	—
1 medium pork chop, lean only, broiled	110	50	50	—
1 slice bologna	85	19.2	76	4.8
1 frankfurter	150	15.7	82.3	2
1 ounce dry salami	135	21.8	77	1.2
DESSERTS, SNACKS, SOFT DRINKS				
¾ cup ice cream	205	7.4	54	38.6
6 ounces cola	65	—	—	100
6 ounces ginger ale	50	—	—	100
⅙ slice of 9-inch apple pie	410	3.4	38.6	58
⅙ slice of 9-inch custard pie	350	11.5	46	42.5
⅙ slice of 9-inch lemon meringue pie	360	6	35	59
1 cup popcorn with oil	70	11.3	38	50.7
10 potato chips	115	3.5	62	34.5
½ cup chocolate pudding	160	10.3	20.7	69

Food	Calories	Percent Protein	Percent Fat	Percent Carbo-hydrate
⅔ cup rice pudding	210	9	20.4	70.6
2-inch piece chocolate cake	370	4.7	37.3	58
1 ounce milk chocolate candy	155	6	53.5	40.5
3 small assorted cookies	120	5	36	59
1 medium doughnut	125	6.5	58	35.5
½ cup Jello	70	62	—	38

Bibliography

General Sources

Allsen, P., J. Harrison and B. Vance. *Fitness for life.* Dubuque: Brown, 1980.

Åstrand, P.-O., and K. Rodahl. *Textbook of work physiology.* New York: McGraw-Hill, 1977.

Beller, A. *Fat and thin.* New York: McGraw-Hill, 1977.

Bennett, W., and J. Gurin. *The dieter's dilemma.* New York: Basic, 1982.

Björntorp, P., M. Cairella and A. Howard (editors). *Recent advances in obesity research: III.* London: John Libbey, 1981.

Bray, G. (editor). *Obesity in America.* National Institutes of Health Publication No. 80-359, 1980.

Bray, G. (editor). *Obesity: Comparative methods of weight control.* Westport, CT: Technomic, 1980.

Bray, G. (editor). *Recent advances in obesity research: II.* Westport, CT: Technomic, 1978.

Brownell, K. *Behavior therapy for weight control.* Philadelphia: University of Pennsylvania, 1979.

Cioffi, L., W. James and T. Van Itallie (editors). *The body weight regulatory system: Normal and disturbed mechanisms.* New York: Raven, 1981.

Collipp, P. (editor). *Childhood obesity,* 2nd ed. Littleton, MA: Wright-PSG, 1980.

de Vries, H. *Physiology of exercise.* Dubuque: W. C. Brown, 1980.

Farquhar, J. *The American way of life need not be hazardous to your health.* New York: W. W. Norton, 1979.

Fixx, J. *The complete book of running.* New York: Random House, 1977.

Fox, E. *Sports physiology.* Philadelphia: Saunders, 1979.

Garrow, J. *Energy balance and obesity in man.* Amsterdam: Elsevier, 1978.

Geliebter, A. Exercise and obesity. In B. Wolman (editor), *Psychological aspects of obesity: A handbook.* New York: Van Nostrand Reinhold, 1982.

Gutin, B. A model of physical fitness and dynamic health. *Journal of physical education and recreation* 51(5):48–51, 1980.

Healthy people: The Surgeon General's report on health promotion and disease prevention. Washington: Department of Health, Education and Welfare, 1979.

Howard, A. (editor). *Recent advances in obesity research: I.* Westport, CT: Technomic, 1974.

Johnson, W., and E. Buskirk (editors). *Science and medicine of exercise and sport.* New York: Harper & Row, 1974.

Johnson, W., and P. Stalonas. *Weight no longer.* Gretna, LA: Pelican, 1981.

Katch, F., and W. McArdle. *Nutrition, weight control, and exercise.* Boston: Houghton Mifflin, 1977.

Lowenthal, D., K. Bharadwaja and W. Oaks (editors). *Therapeutics through exercise.* New York: Grune & Stratton, 1979.

Mayer, J. *Overweight: Causes, cost, and control.* Englewood Cliffs: Prentice-Hall, 1968.

McArdle, W., F. Katch and V. Katch. *Exercise physiology.* Philadelphia: Lea & Febiger, 1981.

Mirkin, G., and M. Hoffman. *The sportsmedicine book.* Boston: Little, Brown, 1978.

Munro, J. (editor). *The treatment of obesity.* Baltimore: University Park Press, 1979.

Nash, J., and L. Long. *Taking charge of your weight and well-being.* Palo Alto: Bull, 1978.

Parizkova, J., and V. Rogozkin (editors). *Nutrition, physical fitness, and health.* Baltimore: University Park Press, 1978.

Rarick, L. (editor) *Physical activity: Human growth and development.* New York: Academic, 1973.

Strauss, R. (editor). *Sports medicine and physiology.* Philadelphia: Saunders, 1979.

Stunkard, A. (editor). *Obesity.* Philadelphia: Saunders, 1980.

Thomas, G., P. Lee, P. Franks and R. Paffenbarger. *Exercise and health.* Cambridge: Oelgeschlager, Gunn and Hain, 1981.

Thompson, J., G. Jarvei, B. Lahey and K. Cureton. Exercise and obesity: Etiology, physiology, and intervention. *Psychological Bulletin* 91 (1): 55–79, 1982.

Zohman, L., A. Kattus and D. Softness. *The cardiologists' guide to fitness and health through exercise.* New York: Simon & Schuster, 1979.

Chapter 1

Belloc, N. Relationship of health practices and mortality. *Preventive Medicine* 2: 67–81, 1973.

Belloc, N., and L. Breslow. The relation of physical health status and health practices. *Preventive Medicine* 1:409–421, 1972.

Berchtold, P., M. Berger, V. Jörgens, C. Daweke, E. Chantelau, F. Gries and H. Zimmerman. Cardiovascular risk factors and HDL-cholesterol levels in obesity. *International Journal of Obesity* 5: 1–10, 1981.

Breslow, L. Research in a strategy for health improvement. *International Journal of Health Services* 3:7–16, 1973.

Keen, H., B. Thomas, R. Jarrett and J. Fuller. Nutrient intake, adiposity, and diabetes. *British Medical Journal* 1:655–658, 1979.

Khosla, T. Obesity, smoking and health. *Community Medicine* 1: 221–228, 1979.

Kraus, H., and W. Raab. *Hypokinetic disease.* Springfield: Thomas, 1961.

Schacter, S. Recidivism and self-cure of smoking and obesity. *American Psychologist* 37:436–444, 1982.

Sorlie, P., T. Gordon and W. Kannel. Body build and mortality. *Journal of the American Medical Association* 243:1828–1831, 1980.

Chapter 2

Berland, T. *Diets '80: Rating the diets.* Skokie, IL: Consumer Guide, 1980.

Bistrian, B. Clinical use of a protein-sparing modified fast. *Journal of the American Medical Association* 240:2299–2302, 1978.

Bogardus, C., B. La Grange, E. Horton and E. Sims. Comparison of carbohydrate-containing and carbohydrate-restricted hypocaloric diets in the treatment of obesity. *Journal of Clinical Investigation* 68:399–404, 1981.

Boyle, P., L. Storlien, A. Harper and R. Keesey. Oxygen consumption and locomotor activity during restricted feeding and realimentation. *American Journal of Physiology* 241:R392–R397, 1981.

Forsum, E., P. Hillman and M. Nesheim. Effect of energy restriction on total heat production, basal metabolic rate, and specific dynamic action of food in rats. *Journal of Nutrition* 111:1691–1697, 1981.

Hirsch, J., and J. Knittle. Cellularity of obese and nonobese human adipose tissue. *Federation Proceedings* 29:1516–1521, 1970.

Isner, J., H. Sours, A. Paris, V. Ferrans and W. Roberts. Sudden, unexpected death in avid dieters using the liquid-protein-modified-fast diet. *Circulation* 60:1401–1412, 1979.

Jung, R., M. Gurr, M. Robinson and W. James. Does adipocyte hypercellularity in obesity exist? *British Medical Journal* 2:319–321, 1978.

Kitsopanides, J., D. Koutras, A. Souvatzoglou, M. Boukis, G. Piperingos, J. Sfontouris and S. Moulopoulos. Metabolic insufficiency as a limiting factor in the dietetic treatment of obesity. *Hormonal and Metabolic Research* 13:477–479, 1981.

Lantigua, R., J. Amatruda, T. Biddle, G. Forbes and D. Lockwood. Cardiac arrhythmias associated with a liquid protein diet for the treatment of obesity. *New England Journal of Medicine* 303:735–738, 1980.

Mirkin, G., and R. Shore. The Beverly Hills diet: Dangers of the newest weight loss fad. *Journal of the American Medical Association* 246:2235–2237, 1981.

Oscai, L. The role of exercise in weight control. In J. Wilmore (editor), *Exercise and sport sciences reviews, volume 1.* New York: Academic, 1973.

Rothwell, N., and M. Stock. Regulation of energy balance. *Annual Review of Nutrition* 1:235–256, 1981.

Stunkard, A., and J. Rush. Dieting and depression reexamined. *Annals of Internal Medicine* 81:526–532, 1974.

Yang, M., and T. Van Itallie. Composition of weight lost during short-term weight reduction. *Journal of Clinical Investigation* 58: 722–730, 1976.

Zahorska-Markiewicz, B. Energy expenditure in obese women on a reducing diet. *Acta Physiologica Polanica* 32:99–102, 1981.

Chapter 3

Belbeck, L., and J. Critz. Effect of exercise on the plasma concentration of anorexigenic substance in man. *Proceedings of the Society for Experimental Biology and Medicine* 142:19–21, 1973.

Björntorp, P. Results of conservative therapy of obesity: Correlation with adipose tissue morphology. *American Journal of Clinical Nutrition* 33:370–375, 1980.

Blair, S., A. Blair, R. Pate, H. Howe, M. Rosenberg and G. Parker. Interactions among dietary pattern, physical activity and skinfold thickness. *Research Quarterly for Exercise and Sport* 52:505–511, 1981.

Blair, S., N. Ellsworth, W. Haskell, M. Stern, J. Farquhar and P. Wood. Comparison of nutrient intake in middle-aged men and women runners and controls. *Medicine and Science in Sports and Exercise* 13:310–315, 1981.

Bloom, W., and M. Eidex. Inactivity as a major factor in adult obesity. *Metabolism* 16:679–684, 1967.

Crews, E., K. Fuge, L. Oscai, J. Holloszy and R. Shank. Weight, food intake, and body composition: Effects of exercise and of protein deficiency. *American Journal of Physiology* 216:275–287, 1969.

Dahlkoetter, J., E. Callahan and J. Linton. Obesity and the unbalanced energy equation: Exercise versus eating habit change. *Journal of Consulting and Clinical Psychology* 47:898–905, 1979.

DeLuise, M., G. Blackburn and J. Flier. Reduced activity of the red-cell sodium-potassium pump in human obesity. *New England Journal of Medicine* 303:1017–1022, 1980.

Gleeson, M., J. Brown, J. Waring and M. Stock. The effects of physical exercise on metabolic rate and dietary-induced thermogenesis. *British Journal of Medicine* 47:173–181, 1982.

Grinker, J., J. Most, J. Hirsch, L. Borsdors and T. Wayler. Long-term follow-up of the effects of a residential weight loss program. *Alimentazione Nutrizione Metabolismo* 1:272, 1980.

Gwinup, G. Effect of exercise alone on the weight of obese women. *Archives of Internal Medicine* 135:676–680, 1975.

Himms-Hagen, J. Obesity may be due to a malfunctioning of brown fat. *Canadian Medical Association Journal* 121:1361–1364, 1979.

Johnson, W., P. Stalonas, M. Christ and S. Pock. The development and evaluation of a behavioral weight-reduction program. *International Journal of Obesity* 3:229–238, 1979.

Katch, F., R. Martin and J. Martin. Effects of exercise intensity on food consumption in the male rat. *American Journal of Clinical Nutrition* 32:1401–1407, 1979.

Leon, A., J. Conrad, D. Hunninghake and R. Serfass. Effects of a vigorous walking program on body composition, and carbohydrate and lipid metabolism of obese young men. *American Journal of Clinical Nutrition* 33:1776–1787, 1979.

Lewis, S., W. Haskell, P. Wood, N. Manoogian, J. Bailey and M. Periera. Effects of physical activity on weight reduction in obese middle-aged women. *American Journal of Clinical Nutrition* 29: 151–156, 1976.

Miller, P., and K. Sims. Evaluation and component analysis of a comprehensive weight control program. *International Journal of Obesity* 5:57–65, 1981.

Mir, M., B. Charalambous, K. Morgan and P. Evans. Erythrocyte sodium-potassium ATPase and sodium transport in obesity. *New England Journal of Medicine* 305:1264–1268, 1981.

Mohr, D. Changes in waistline and abdominal girth and subcutaneous fat following isometric exercises. *Research Quarterly* 36:169–173, 1965.

Moody, D., J. Kollias and E. Buskirk. The effect of a moderate exercise program on body weight and skinfold thickness in overweight college women. *Medicine and Science in Sports* 1:75–80, 1969.

Newsholme, E. A possible metabolic basis for the control of body weight. *New England Journal of Medicine* 302:400–405, 1980.

Norgan, N., and J. Durnin. The effect of six weeks of overfeeding on the body weight, body composition, and energy metabolism of young men. *American Journal of Clinical Nutrition* 33:978–988, 1980.

O'Hara, W., C. Allen and R. Shephard. Loss of body weight and fat during exercise in a cold chamber. *European Journal of Applied Physiology* 37:205–218, 1977,

O'Hara, W., C. Allen and R. Shephard. Loss of body fat during an arctic winter expedition. *Canadian Journal of Physiology and Pharmacology* 55:1235–1241, 1977.

Olson, A., and E. Edelstein. Spot reduction of subcutaneous adipose tissue. *Research Quarterly* 39:647–652, 1968.

Oscai, L., and J. Holloszy. Effects of weight changed produced by exercise, food restriction, or overeating on body composition. *Journal of Clinical Investigation* 48:2124–2128, 1969.

Oscai, L., and J. Holloszy. Weight reduction in obese rats by exercise or food restriction: Effect on the heart. *American Journal of Physiology* 219:327–330, 1970.

Oscai, L., C. Spirakis, C. Wolff and R. Beck. Effects of exercise and of food restriction on adipose tissue cellularity. *Journal of Lipid Research* 13:588–592, 1972.

Peterson, J., and T. Brigham. Women, weight loss, and working out: The effects of exercise on weight control. Presented at meeting of the Association for the Advancement of Behavior Therapy, New York, 1980.

Pitts, G., and L. Bull. Exercise, dietary obesity, and growth in the rat. *American Journal of Physiology* 232:R38–R44, 1977.

Rothwell, N., and M. Stock. A role for brown adipose tissue in diet-induced thermogenesis. *Nature* 281:31–35, 1979.

Salans, L., E. Horton and E. Sims. Experimental obesity in man: Cellular character of the adipose tissue. *Journal of Clinical Investigation* 50:1005–1011, 1971.

Shetty, P., R. Jung, W. James, M. Barrand and B. Callingham. Postprandial thermogenesis in obesity. *Clinical Science* 60:519–525, 1981.

Segal, K. and B. Gutin. Thermic effects of food and exercise in lean and obese women. *American Journal of Clinical Nutrition* 35:xvi, 1982.

Simko, V., H. Merrifield and J. Stouffer. Mild exercise: Effect on body composition and metabolism. *New York State Journal of Medicine* 74:1563–1567, 1974.

Stalonas, P., W. Johnson and M. Christ. Behavior modification for obesity: The evaluation of exercise, contingency management, and program adherence. *Journal of Consulting and Clinical Psychology* 46:463–469, 1978.

Stern, J., C. Schultz, P. Molé, H. Superko and E. Bernauer. Effect of caloric restriction and exercise on basal metabolism and thyroid hormone. *Alimentazione Nutrizione Metabolismo, Vol. 1.* From Third International Congress on Obesity, Rome, 1980.

Woo, R., J. Garrow and F. X. Pi-Sunyer. Effect of exercise on spontaneous calorie intake in obesity. *American Journal of Clinical Nutrition* 36:470–477, 1982.

Woo, R., J. Garrow and F. X. Pi-Sunyer. Voluntary food intake during prolonged exercise in obese women. *American Journal of Clinical Nutrition* 36:478–484, 1982.

Zuti, W., and L. Golding. Comparing diet and exercise as weight reduction tools. *The Physician and Sportsmedicine* 4(1):49–53, 1976.

Chapter 4

Cooper, K. *Aerobics.* New York: Bantam, 1968.

Enelow, A., and J. Henderson (editors). *Applying behavioral science to cardiovascular risk.* American Heart Association, 1975.

Konishi, F., J. Kesselman and F. Peterson. *Eat anything exercise diet.* New York: Morrow, 1979.

Watson, D., and R. Tharp. *Self-directed behavior.* Monterey: Brooks/Cole, 1977.

Chapter 5

American College of Sports Medicine. Position Statement: The recommended quantity and quality of exercise for developing and maintaining fitness in healthy adults. *Medicine and Science in Sports* 10:vii–x, 1978.

Cooper, K. *The new aerobics.* New York: Bantam, 1970.

Davis, J., M. Frank, B. Whipp and K. Wasserman. Anaerobic threshold alterations caused by endurance training in middle-aged men. *Journal of Applied Physiology* 46:1039–1046, 1979.

Delza, S. *Tai chi ch'uan.* New York: Cornerstone, 1974.

Gettman, L., M. Pollock, J. Durstine, A. Ward, J. Ayres and A. Linnerud. Physiological responses of men to 1, 3, and 5 day per week training programs. *Research Quarterly* 47:638–646, 1976.

Gutin, B., and S. Lipetz. An electromyographic investigation of the rectus abdominis in various abdominal exercises. *Research Quarterly* 42:256–263, 1971.

Gutin, B., J. Young, J. Simon, D. Blood and G. Dixon. Anaerobic threshold as determined by plasma lactate, ventilatory indices, and perceived discomfort. *Medicine and Science in Sports and Exercise* 12: 124, 1980.

Gutin, B., K. Torrey, R. Welles and M. Vytvytski. Physiological parameters related to running performance in college trackmen. *Journal of Human Ergology* 4:27–34, 1975.

Gutin, B., A. Trinidad, C. Norton, E. Giles, K. Stewart and A. Giles. Morphological and physiological factors related to endurance performance of eleven- to twelve-year-old girls. *Research Quarterly* 49:44–52, 1978.

Hickson, R., H. Bomze and J. Holloszy. Linear increase in aerobic power induced by a strenuous program of endurance exercise. *Journal of Applied Physiology* 42:372–376, 1977.

Igbanugo, V., and B. Gutin. The energy cost of aerobic dancing. *Research Quarterly* 49: 308–316, 1978.

Katz, J. *Swimming for total fitness.* Garden City: Dolphin, 1981.

Kraus, H. *The causes, prevention and treatment of sports injuries.* New York: Playboy Press, 1981.

Leger, L. Energy cost of disco dancing. *Research Quarterly for Exercise and Sport* 53: 46–49, 1982.

Lipetz, S., and B. Gutin. An electromyographic study of four abdominal exercises. *Medicine and Science in Sports* 2: 35–38, 1970.

Mayers, N., and B. Gutin. Physiological characteristics of elite prepubertal cross country runners. *Medicine and Science in Sports* 11: 172–176, 1979.

Palgi, Y., B. Gutin, J. Young and D. Alejandro. Physiological and anthropometric factors underlying endurance in children. *Medicine and Science in Sports and Exercise* 12:143, 1980.

Simon, J., B. Gutin, J. Young and D. Blood. Lactate accumulation during constant work load just below and just above the anaerobic and respiratory compensation thresholds. *Medicine and Science in Sports and Exercise* 12:126, 1980.

Stewart, K., and B. Gutin. Effects of physical training on cardiorespiratory fitness in children. *Research Quarterly* 47:110–120, 1976.

Torrey, K., J. Young and B. Gutin. The effects of interval and continuous aerobic training on submaximal and maximal exercise response, and endurance performance in college aged males. Presented at meeting of Greater New York Chapter of the American College of Sports Medicine, 1980.

Wasserman, K., B. Whipp, S. Koyal and W. Beaver. Anaerobic threshold and respiratory gas exchange during exercise. *Journal of Applied Physiology* 35:236–243, 1973.

Weltman, A., V. Katch, S. Sady and P. Freedson. Onset of metabolic acidosis (anaerobic threshold) as a criterion measure of submaximum fitness. *Research Quarterly* 49:218–227, 1978.

Young, J., B. Gutin, J. Simon, G. Dixon and D. Alejandro. Non-invasive assessment of the anaerobic threshold. Presented at Greater New York Chapter of the American College of Sports Medicine, 1978.

Chapter 6

American College of Sports Medicine. *Guidelines for graded exercise testing and exercise prescription.* Philadelphia: Lea & Febiger, 1980.

American Heart Association. *A guide to prevention and treatment of cardiovascular diseases.* New York: American Heart Association, 1980.

Andzel, W., and B. Gutin. Prior exercise and endurance performance: a test of the mobilization hypothesis. *Research Quarterly* 47:269–276, 1976.

Barnard, R., G. Gardner, N. Diaco, R. MacAlpin and A. Kattus. Cardiovascular responses to sudden strenuous exercise—heart rate, blood pressure, and ECG. *Journal of Applied Physiology* 34:833–837, 1973.

Chung, E. *Exercise electrocardiography.* Baltimore: Williams and Wilkins, 1979.

Ellestad, M. *Stress testing.* Philadelphia: Davis, 1980.

Gutin, B. Exercise-induced activation and human performance: a review. *Research Quarterly* 44:256–268, 1973.

Gutin, B., R. Fogle, J. Meyer and M. Jaeger. Steadiness as a function of prior exercise. *Journal of Motor Behavior* 6:69–76, 1974.

Gutin, B., K. Stewart, S. Lewis and J. Kruper. Oxygen consumption in the first stages of strenuous work as a function of prior exercise. *Journal of Sports Medicine and Physical Fitness* 16:60–65, 1976.

Gutin, B., J. Wilkerson, S. Horvath and R. Rochelle. Physiologic response to endurance work as a function of prior exercise. *International Journal of Sports Medicine* 2:87–91, 1981.

National Heart, Lung and Blood Institute. *Exercise and your heart.* Bethesda: NIH, 1981.

Chapter 7

Adamovich, D., D. Lubell and B. Gutin. Systolic time intervals as a function of posture, exercise intensity and cardiac status. *Proceedings of International Conference on Sports Cardiology.* Bologna: Aulo Gaggi, 1978.

Amsterdam, E., J. Wilmore and A. DeMaria (editors). *Exercise in cardiovascular health and disease.* New York: Yorke Medical, 1977.

Benson, H. *The relaxation response.* New York: Avon, 1976.

Björntorp, P., M. Fahlén, G. Grimby, A. Gustafson, J. Holm, P. Renström and T. Schersten. Carbohydrate and lipid metabolism in middle-aged physically well-trained men. *Metabolism* 21:1037, 1972.

Blanding, F. *The pulse point plan.* New York: Random House, 1982.

Brownell, K., and A. Stunkard. Differential changes in plasma high-density-lipoprotein-cholesterol levels in obese men and women during weight reduction. *Archives of Internal Medicine* 141:1142–1146, 1981.

Brownell, K., P. Bachorik and R. Ayerle. Changes in plasma lipid and lipoprotein levels in men and women after a program of moderate exercise. *Circulation* 65:477–484, 1982.

Carrington, P., G. Collings, Jr., H. Benson, H. Robinson, L. Wood, P. Lehrer, R. Woolfolk and J. Cole. The use of meditation-relaxation techniques for the management of stress in a working population. *Journal of Occupational Medicine* 22:221–231, 1980.

Cooper, K., M. Pollock, R. Martin, S. White, A. Linnerud and A. Jackson. Physical fitness levels vs. selected coronary risk factors. *Journal of the American Medical Association* 236:166–169, 1976.

de Vries, H. Tranquilizer effect of exercise: A critical review. *The Physician and Sportsmedicine* 9(11):47–55, 1981.

Friedman, M. Type A behavior: A progress report. *The Sciences,* February 1980.

Fusco, R., and B. Gutin. Effects of exercise training on cardiovascular response of human subjects to a localized cold stressor. *American Corrective Therapy Journal* 28:42–46, 1974.

Goodrick, C. Effects of long-term voluntary wheel exercise on male and female Wistar rats. *Gerontology* 26:22–33, 1980.

Gordon, T., W. Castelli, M. Hjortland, W. Kannel and T. Dawber. High density lipoprotein as a protective factor against coronary heart disease. *American Journal of Medicine* 62:707–714, 1977.

Gutin, B., L. Zohman and J. Young. Case report of an eighty-year-old marathoner. *Journal of Cardiac Rehabilitation* 1:344–348, 1981.

Hannum, S., and F. Kasch. Acute postexercise blood pressure response of hypertensive and normotensive men. *Scandinavian Journal of Sport Sciences* 3:11–15, 1981.

Hartung, G., J. Foreyt, R. Mitchell, I. Vlasek and A. Gotto. Relation of diet to high-density-lipoprotein cholesterol in middle-aged marathon runners, joggers and inactive men. *New England Journal of Medicine* 302:357–361, 1980.

Heath, G., J. Hagberg, A. Ehsani and J. Holloszy. A physiological comparison of young and older endurance athletes. *Journal of Applied Physiology* 51:634–640, 1981.

Hoffman, J., H. Benson, P. Arns, G. Stainbrook, L. Landsberg, J. Young and A. Gill. Reduced sympathetic nervous system responsivity associated with the relaxation response. *Science* 215:190–192, 1982.

Jacobson, E. *You must relax.* New York: McGraw-Hill, 1962.

Kannel, W., and D. McGee. Diabetes and glucose tolerance as risk factors for cardiovascular disease: The Framingham study. *Diabetes Care* 2:120–126, 1979.

Kasch, F., and J. Kulberg. Physiological variables during fifteen years of endurance exercise. *Scandinavian Journal of Sports Sciences* 3: 59–62, 1981.

Keys, A. Is overweight a risk factor of coronary heart disease? *Cardiovascular Medicine* 4(12):1233–1243, 1979.

Kissebah, A., N. Vydelingum, R. Murray, D. Evans, A. Hartz, R. Kalkhoff and P. Adams. Relation of body fat distribution to metabolic complications of obesity. *Journal of Clinical Endocrinology and Metabolism* 54:254–259, 1982.

Kluger, M., and J. Cannon. Running a fever. Brief report in *The Sciences,* August/September, 1982.

Kramsch, D., A. Aspen, B. Abramowitz, T. Kreimendahl and W.

Hood. Reduction of coronary atherosclerosis by moderate conditioning exercise in monkeys on an atherogenic diet. *New England Journal of Medicine* 305:1483–1484, 1981.

Kraus, H. *The cause, prevention and treatment of backache, stress and tension.* New York: Pocket, 1965.

Kraus, H. *Clinical treatment of back pain.* New York: McGraw-Hill, 1970.

Morris, J., R. Pollard, M. Everitt, S. Chave and A. Semmence. Vigorous exercise in leisure time: Protection against coronary heart disease. *The Lancet,* December 6, 1980.

Orth-Gomer, K., and A. Ahlbom. Impact of psychological stress on ischemic heart disease when controlling for conventional risk indicators. *Journal of Human Stress,* March 1980.

Paffenbarger, R., A. Wing and R. Hyde. Physical activity as an index of heart attack risk in college alumni. *American Journal of Epidemiology* 108:161–175, 1978.

Paffenberger, R., W. Hale, R. Brand and R. Hyde. Work-energy level, personal characteristics, and fatal heart attack: A birth-cohort effect. *American Journal of Epidemiology* 105:200–213, 1977.

Peltonen, P., J. Marniemi, E. Hietanen, I. Vuori and C. Ehnholm. Changes in serum lipids, lipoproteins, and heparin releasable lipolytic enzymes during moderate physical training in man: a longitudinal study. *Metabolism* 30:518–526, 1981.

Persky, V., A. Dyer, J. Leonas, J. Stamler, D. Berkson, H. Lindberg, O. Paul, R. Shekelle, M. Lepper and J. Schoenberger. Heart rate: A risk factor for cancer? *American Journal of Epidemiology* 114: 477–487, 1981.

Pollock, M., and D. Schmidt (editors). *Heart disease and rehabilitation.* Boston: Houghton-Mifflin, 1979.

Raab, W. (editor). *Prevention of ischemic heart disease.* Springfield, IL: Thomas, 1966.

Retzlaff, E., J. Fontaine and W. Furuta. Effect of daily exercise on life-span of albino rats. *Geriatrics,* March 1966, pp. 171–177.

Shephard, R. *Physical activity and aging.* Chicago: Year Book Medical, 1978.

Shephard, R. *Ischaemic heart disease and exercise.* Chicago: Year Book Medical, 1981.

Smith, E., and R. Serfass (editors). *Exercise and aging.* Hillside, NJ: Enslow, 1981.

Smith, E. Exercise for prevention of osteoporosis: A review. *The Physician and Sportsmedicine* 10(3):72–80, 1982.

Smith, E., W. Reddan and P. Smith. Physical activity and calcium modalities for bone mineral increase in aged women. *Medicine and Science in Sports and Exercise* 13:60–64, 1981.

Streja, D., E. Boyco and S. Rabkin. Changes in plasma high-density lipoprotein cholesterol concentration after weight reduction in grossly obese subjects. *British Medical Journal* 281:770–772, 1980.

Weindruch, R., and R. Walford. Dietary restriction in mice beginning at one year of age: effect on life-span and spontaneous cancer incidence. *Science* 215:1415–1417, 1982.

Weltman, A., S. Matter and B. Stamford. Caloric restriction and/or mild exercise: Effects on serum lipids and body composition. *American Journal of Clinical Nutrition* 33:1002–1009, 1980.

Wolinsky, H. Taking heart. *The Sciences,* February 1981.

Wood, P., W. Haskell, M. Stern, S. Lewis, and C. Perry. Plasma lipoprotein distributions in male and female runners. *Annals of the New York Academy of Sciences* 301:748–763, 1977.

Wood, P., and W. Haskell. The effect of exercise on plasma high density lipoproteins. *Lipids* 14:417–427, 1979.

Zavaroni, I., Y. Chen, C. Mondon and G. Reaven. Ability of exercise to inhibit carbohydrate-induced hypertriglyceridemia in rats. *Metabolism* 30:476–480.

Zimkin, N. Stress during muscular exercises and the state of nonspecifically increased resistance. In E. Jokl and E. Simon (editors), *International research in physical education.* Springfield, IL: Thomas, 1964.

Chapter 8

Benson, H., T. Dryer and L. Hartley. Decreased oxygen consumption during exercise with elicitation of the relaxation response. *Journal of Human Stress* 4:38–42, 1978.

Berger, B., and D. Owen. The positive effects of swimming on mood:

Swimmers really do feel better. Presented at conference of North American Society for the Psychology of Sport and Physical Activity, College Park, MD, 1982.

Bortz, W., P. Angwin, I. Mafford, M. Boarder, N. Noyce, and J. Barchas. Catecholamines, dopamine, and endorphin levels during extreme exercise. *New England Journal of Medicine* 305:466–467, 1981.

Brown, R., D. Ramirez and J. Taub. The prescription of exercise for depression. *The Physician and Sportsmedicine* 6(12):34–45, 1978.

Collingwood, T. Effective physical functioning: A precondition for the helping process. *Counselor Education and Supervision,* March 1976.

deVries, H. *Vigor regained.* Englewood Cliffs: Prentice-Hall, 1974.

Folkins, C. Effects of physical training on mood. *Journal of Clinical Psychology* 32:385–388, 1976.

Folkins, C., and W. Sime. Physical fitness training and mental health. *American Psychologist* 36:373–389, 1981.

Fraioli, F., C. Moretti, D. Paolucci, E. Alicicco, F. Crescenzi and G. Fortunio. Physical exercise stimulates marked concomitant release of B-endorphin and adrenocorticotropic hormone (ACTH) in peripheral blood in man. *Experientia* 36:987–988, 1980.

Gambert, S., T. Garthwaite, C. Pontzer, E. Cook, F. Tristani, E. Duthie, D. Martinson, T. Hagen and D. McCarty. Running elevates plasma B-endorphin immunoreactivity and ACTH in untrained human subjects. *Proceedings of the Society for Experimental Biology and Medicine* 168:1–4, 1981.

Glasser, W. *Positive addiction.* New York: Harper and Row, 1976.

Greist, J., R. Eischens, M. Klein and J. Faris. Antidepressant running. *Psychiatric Annals* 9(3):23–33, 1979.

Harris, D. Physical activity history and attitudes of middle-aged men. *Medicine and Science in Sports* 2:203–208, 1970.

Kostrubala, T. *The joy of running.* New York: Pocket, 1977.

Little, J. Neurotic illness in fitness fanatics. *Psychiatric Annals* 9(3): 49–56, 1979.

Markoff, R., P. Ryan and T. Young. Endorphins and mood changes in long-distance running. *Medicine and Science in Sports and Exercise* 14:11–15, 1982.

Moore, M. Endorphins and exercise: A puzzling relationship. *The Physician and Sportsmedicine* 10(2):111–114, 1982.

Morgan, W. Negative addiction in runners. *The Physician and Sportsmedicine* 7(2):56–70, 1979.

Morgan, W. Anxiety reduction following acute physical activity. *Psychiatric Annals* 9(3):34–45, 1979.

Pargman, D. The way of the runner: An examination of motives for running. In R. Suinn (editor), *Psychology in sports: Methods and applications.* Minneapolis: Burgess, 1980.

Pargman, D., and M. Baker. Running high: Enkephalin indicted. *Journal of Drug Issues,* Summer 1980

Ransford, C. A role for amines in the antidepressant effect of exercise: A review. *Medicine and Science in Sports and Exercise* 14:1–10, 1982.

Sacks, M. A psychodynamic overview of sport. *Psychiatric Annals* 9(3):13–22, 1979.

Sacks, M., and M. Sachs (editors). *Psychology of running.* Champaign, IL: Human Kinetics, 1981.

Sheehan, G. *Running and being.* New York: Simon & Schuster, 1978.

Sheehan, G. Various columns in *The Physician and Sportsmedicine* and *Runner's World.*

Wertheimer, R. Some fast steps to mental fitness. *The Bergen Record,* July 2, 1981.

Chapter 9

Acheson, K., B. Zahorska-Markiewicz, Ph. Pittet, K. Anantharaman and E. Jequier. Caffeine and coffee: Their influence on metabolic rate and substrate utilization in normal weight and obese individuals. *American Journal of Clinical Nutrition* 33:989–997, 1980.

Adams, C. *Nutritive value of American foods.* Washington: Agriculture Handbook No. 456, 1975.

Anderson, J., F. Grande and A. Keys. Cholesterol-lowering diets. *Journal of the American Dietetic Association* 62:133–142, 1973.

Asp, N., H. Bauer, P. Nilsson-Ehle, M. Nyman and R. Oste. Wheat bran increases high-density-lipoprotein cholesterol in the rat. *British Journal of Nutrition* 46:385, 1981.

Bogert, L. J., G. Briggs and D. Calloway. *Nutrition and physical fitness.* Philadelphia: W. B. Saunders, 1973.

Brody, J. *Jane Brody's nutrition book.* New York: Norton, 1981.

Buskirk, E. Some nutritional considerations in the conditioning of athletes. *Annual Review of Nutrition* 1:319–350, 1981.

Committee on Diet, Nutrition, and Cancer of National Research Council. *Diet, Nutrition, and Cancer.* Washington: National Academy Press, 1982.

Costill, D., and J. Miller. Nutrition for endurance sport: Carbohydrate and fluid balance. *International Journal of Sports Medicine* 1:2–14, 1980.

Darby, W. The benefits of drink. *Human Nature* 1(11):30–37, 1978.

Davidson, S., R. Passmore, J. Brock and A. Truswell. *Human nutrition and dietetics.* Edinburgh: Churchill Livingstone, 1979.

Ellwood, K., and O. Michaelis. Effects of feeding dietary carbohydrates and cholesterol on blood lipid, insulin, glucose and liver enzymes of Wister rates. *Nutrition Reports International* 24(4): 675–688, 1981.

Food and Nutrition Board, National Research Council, National Academy of Sciences. Toward healthful diets. *Nutrition Today,* May/June 1980.

Fraser, G., and R. Swannell. Diet and serum cholesterol in Seventh-Day Adventists: A cross-sectional study showing significant relationships. *Journal of Chronic Diseases* 34:487–501, 1981.

Hjermann, I., I. Holme, K. Velve Byre and P. Leren. Effect of diet and smoking intervention on the incidence of coronary heart disease. *The Lancet,* December 12, 1981.

Hubbard, R., M. Mager, W. Bowers, I. Leav, G. Angoff, W. Matthew and I. Sils. Effect of low-potassium diet on rat exercise hyperthermia and heatstroke mortality. *Journal of Applied Physiology* 51:8–13, 1981.

Lewis, S., and B. Gutin. Nutrition and endurance. *American Journal of Clinical Nutrition* 26:1011–1014, 1973.

Lewis, B., M. Katan, I. Merkx, N. Miller, F. Hammett, R. Kay, A. Nobels and A. Swan. Towards an improved lipid-lowering diet:

Additive effects of changes in nutrient intake. *The Lancet,* December 12, 1981.

Malhotra, K. Sridharan, Y. Ventkaswamy, R. Rai, G. Pichan, U. Radkakrishnan and S. Grover. Effect of restricted potassium intake on its excretion and on physiological responses during heat stress. *European Journal of Applied Physiology* 47:169–179, 1981.

Morgan, G. Alcohol as a health hazard. *Nutrition and Health* 3(3): 1–6, 1981.

Nelson, R. Nutrition and physical performance. *The Physician and Sportsmedicine* 10(4):55–63, 1982.

Nuttall, F. Dietary recommendations for individuals with diabetes mellitus, 1979: Summary of report from the Food and Nutrition Committee of the American Diabetes Association. *American Journal of Clinical Nutrition* 33:1311–1312, 1980.

Roberts, S., M. McMurry and W. Connor. Does egg feeding (i.e. dietary cholesterol) affect plasma cholesterol levels in humans? The results of a double-blind study. *American Journal of Clinical Nutrition* 34:2092–2099, 1981.

Rockstein, M., and M. Sussman (editors). *Nutrition, longevity and aging.* New York: Academic, 1976.

Rudle, L., C. Leathers, M. Bond and B. Bullock. Dietary ethanol-induced modifications in hyperlipoproteinemia and atherosclerosis in nonhuman primates (Macaca nemistrina). *Atherosclerosis* 1: 144–155, 1981.

Sacks, F., A. Donner, W. Castelli, J. Gronemeyer, P. Pletka, H. Margolius, L. Landsberg, and E. Kass. Effect of ingestion of meat on plasma cholesterol of vegetarians. *Journal of the American Medical Association* 246: 640–644, 1981.

Saltin, B. Metabolic fundamentals in exercise. *Medicine and Science in Sports* 5:137–146, 1973.

Select Committee on Nutrition and Human Needs, United States Senate. *Dietary goals for the United States.* Washington: U.S. Government Printing Office, 1977.

Simpson, H., S. Lousley, M. Geekie, R. Simpson, R. Carter, T. Hockeday and J. Mann. A high carbohydrate leguminous fibre diet improves all aspects of diabetic control. *The Lancet,* January 3, 1981.

Smith, N. *Food for sport.* Palo Alto: Bull, 1976.

Torun, B., N. Scrimshaw and V. Young. Effect of isometric exercises on body potassium and dietary protein requirements of young men. *American Journal of Clinical Nutrition* 30:1983–1993, 1977.

Watt, B., and A. Merrill. *Composition of foods.* Washington: Agriculture Handbook No. 8, 1975.

Winick, M. Diet and the cause of cancer. *Nutrition and Health* 1(5): 1–6, 1979.

Winick, M. Diet and the risk of "heart attack." *Nutrition and Health* 1(1):1–6, 1979.

Zauner, C., J. Burt and D. Mapes. Effect of strenuous and mild pre-meal exercise on postprandial lipemia. *Research Quarterly* 39: 395–401, 1968.

Chapter 10

Biermann, J., and B. Toohey. *The diabetic's sports and exercise book.* New York: Lippincott, 1977.

Björntorp, P. Results of conservative therapy of obesity: Correlation with adipose tissue morphology. *American Journal of Clinical Nutrition* 33:370–375, 1980.

Cohen, J., C. Kim, P. May and N. Ertel. Exercise, body weight, and amenorrhea in professional ballet dancers. *The Physician and Sportsmedicine* 10(4):92–101, 1982.

Dressendorfer, R. Physical training during pregnancy and lactation. *The Physician and Sportsmedicine* 6(2):74–80, 1978.

Ehsani, A., G. Heath, J. Hagberg, B. Sobel and J. Holloszy. Effects of 12 months of intense exercise training on ischemic ST-segment depression in patients with coronary artery disease. *Circulation* 64:1116–1124, 1981.

Engerbretson, D. The diabetic in physical education, recreation and athletics. *Journal of Physical Education and Recreation,* March 1977.

Frisch, R. Fatness, puberty, and fertility. *Natural History* 89(10): 22–27, 1980.

Frisch, R., G. Wyshak and L. Vincent. Delayed menarche and amenorrhea in ballet dancers. *New England Journal of Medicine* 303: 17–19, 1980.

Gilliam, T., S. MacConnie, D. Geenen, A. Pels and P. Freedson. Exercise programs for children: A way to prevent heart disease? *The Physician and Sportsmedicine* 10(9):96–108, 1982.

Gordon, T., W. Castelli, M. Hjortland, W. Kannel and T. Dawber. Diabetes, blood lipids and the role of obesity in coronary heart disease risk for women. *Annals of Internal Medicine* 87:393–397, 1977.

Hoffman, W. The effect of propranolol on change in HDL level in cardiac patients involved in exercise training. *Medicine and Science in Sports and Exercise* 14:124, 1982.

Krotkiewski, M., K. Mandroukas, L. Sjöström, L. Sullivan, H. Wellerqvist, and P. Björntorp. Effects of long-term physical training on body fat, metabolism, and blood pressure in obesity. *Metabolism* 28:650–658, 1978.

LeBlanc, J., A. Nadeau, D. Richard, and A. Tremblay. Studies on the sparing effect of exercise on insulin requirements in human subjects. *Metabolism* 30:1119–1124, 1981.

Lohmann, D., F. Liebold, W. Heilmann, H. Senger and A. Pohl. Diminished insulin response in highly trained athletes. *Metabolism* 27:521, 1978.

Chapter 11

Bowne, D. Physical fitness programs for industry—an extravagance or a wise investment? *Transactions of the Association of Life Insurance Medical Directors of America* 64:210–222, 1980.

Brownell, K., and F. Kaye. A school-based behavior modification, nutrition education, and physical activity program for obese children. *American Journal of Clinical Nutrition* 35:277–283, 1982.

Index

exercise programs (*cont.*)
  individualized, 39
  monitoring progress in, 42
  for obese people, 151–53
  physical examination before,
    76–77, 151
exerciser's high, 113–15

fainting, prevention of, 75–76
fasting, 20–21
fat, body:
  in adult-onset vs. childhood-
    onset obesity, 94
  aerobic endurance and, 57
  measurement of, 67–68
  sex differences in, 147
fat, dietary, 120–24
fat cells, 17, 31–34
fatigue:
  anaerobic energy release and,
    51, 54
  exercise and, 45, 47, 54
  injury and, 57
  lactic acid and, 54, 56
  low-carbohydrate diet and, 19
fat-soluble vitamins, 121
fatty acids, essential, 121–22
fiber, dietary, 124–26
fish, 118–19, 120
flexibility, 65–67
  age and, 103
  back pain and, 67
  exercises for, 66, 70
  heredity and, 67
  pain and loss of, 65, 67
Frisch, Rose, 149

fructose, 124
fruits and fruit juices, 140
Fusco, Ronald, 86

Garrow, John, 25
Gettis, Alan, 110
Glasser, William, 114
glucose, 124, 139
glycogen:
  aerobic exercise and, 57
  carbohydrate loading and,
    133–35
  carbohydrate stored as, 121
  water stored with, 46
Godfrey, Simon, 162
Golding, Lawrence, 34
gradualism, principle of, 71–72
Greist, John, 108–9
Grinker, Joel, 35

hamburgers, 130
Hansen, O., 133
Harris, Dorothy, 112
heart disease, *see* coronary heart
  disease
heart patients, exercise program
  for, 156–58
heart rate:
  exercise and, 97
  maximal, 62
heart-rate method, 62
heart-rate response, 58–61
heat cramps, 80
heat exhaustion, 80
Heath, G. W., 102
heatstroke, 80

ABOUT THE AUTHORS

BERNARD GUTIN, Ph.D., is professor of applied physiology and education at Teachers College, Columbia University, and director of physiology of the Weight Control Center at Holy Name Hospital in Teaneck, New Jersey. Dr. Gutin is president of the Greater New York Chapter of the American College of Sports Medicine and a member of the Exercise Committee of the New York Heart Association. His research and clinical work concerns the interactions between exercise and nutrition, as applied to weight control and cardiovascular health. Dr. Gutin lives in New York City, is married and has two children.

GAIL KESSLER has a Ph.D. in English literature from Columbia University, and taught on the high school and college level before becoming a freelance writer. She has published articles in many national magazines, and is the author of *Judgment: A Case of Medical Malpractice* (Mason-Charter, 1976) and *How to Marry a Good Man* (Putnam, 1983). She lives in New Jersey with her husband and two children.